INFORMATION
SYSTEMS
INNOVATIONS
FOR
NURSING

SONA

SERIES ON NURSING ADMINISTRATION

An annual publication planned and administered by the University of Iowa, SONA addresses current and emerging issues in nursing administration. In each volume, distinguished nurse administrators and educators address the state of knowledge, future directions, and controversial questions on aspects of a particular issue and propose options for resolution. The series provides a quality resource for practicing administrators, faculty teaching nursing administration, and students in administration programs.

INFORMATION SYSTEMS INNOVATIONS FOR NURSING

New Visions and Ventures

Edited by
Sue Moorhead
Connie Delaney

Chair of the Board
Diane Huber

SONA Series on Nursing Administration

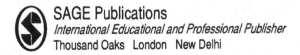

SAGE Publications
International Educational and Professional Publisher
Thousand Oaks   London   New Delhi

For information:

SAGE Publications, Inc.
2455 Teller Road
Thousand Oaks, California 91320
E-mail: order@sagepub.com

SAGE Publications Ltd.
6 Bonhill Street
London EC2A 4PU
United Kingdom

SAGE Publications India Pvt. Ltd.
M-32 Market
Greater Kailash I
New Delhi 110 048 India

Library of Congress Cataloging-in-Publication Data

Information systems innovations for nursing: New visions and
ventures / edited by Sue A. Moorhead and Connie Delaney.
    p. cm. -- (Series on nursing administration ; v. 10)
  Includes bibliographical references and index.
  ISBN 0-7619-1670-9 (cloth : acid-free paper)
  ISBN 0-7619-1671-7 (pbk. : acid-free paper)
  1. Information storage and retrieval systems--Nursing. 2.
Nursing--Data processing. 3. Nursing services--Administration--Data
processing. I. Moorhead, Sue. II. Delaney, Connie White. III.
Series.
  RT50.5 .I55 1998
  610.73'0285--ddc21
                                                              98-9026

This book is printed on acid-free paper.
98 99 00 01 02 03 04 10 9 8 7 6 5 4 3 2 1

Acquisition Editor:	Dan Ruth
Editorial Assistant:	Anna Howland
Production Editor:	Sanford Robinson
Production Assistant:	Karen Wiley
Typesetter/Designer:	Rose Tylak
Cover Designer:	Ravi Balasuriya
Indexer:	Teri Greenberg

Contents

Series Preface

Today's nurse executive needs to stay current in many rapidly changing areas of health care. To meet this demand, the **Series on Nursing Administration** is designed to give nursing administrators new information on current and emerging issues. Developed and managed at the University of Iowa College of Nursing and published by Sage Publications, Inc., it is a quality resource for nurse executives, faculty who teach nursing administration, and students in nursing administration programs. Each volume addresses the most recent issues in this discipline to keep readers on the forefront of knowledge and practice.

Every nurse executive interacts with corporate management, colleagues in other settings, professional groups, the community, and clients; and with nurse colleagues, members of other disciplines, and ancillary personnel. To stay current with developments in each of these areas the nurse executive reads journals and newsletters, attends continuing education programs, and participates in short-term executive management courses. The most effective method, however, is the sharing of concerns, experiences, and insights with peers. The Sage **Series on Nursing Administration** formalizes the process of sharing among experts with similar concerns. In every chapter of each volume of the series, expert authors share their experiences and ideas on particular emerging issues. Busy nurse executives can conveniently and cost-effectively keep their knowledge current on a variety of topics by reading this series.

Nursing administration faculty can use the series to keep their teaching and practice alive, current, and timely. Most nursing administration programs have one or more courses that address issues in nursing management. Because these issues undergo rapid change, faculty need a flexible approach to teaching this content. This series offers the instructor maximum flexibility in selecting issues for discussion to fit the needs of a particular class. An instructor teaching a nursing management issues course can use the series as a course text. Students introduced to this series will find it a resource with ongoing value. Faculty teaching undergraduate-level administration courses also may use the Series to supplement an introductory text on management and leadership.

The series is unique in that it is the first annual series devoted to issues in nursing administration. To ensure that it covers current issues and provides up-to-date information, the series employs a unique publication process involving four groups: a Series editor, an editorial board, the authors, and the publisher.

The editor of Volumes 1 through 4 of the series was Marion Johnson, RN, PhD, an associate professor at the University of Iowa. She has a rich practice base in nursing administration and currently teaches nursing administration at the master's level. Her background, interests, and writing skills made her eminently qualified for the job of series editor.

The late Kathleen Kelly, PhD, RN, was the editor for Volumes 5 through 8 of the series. Kathleen had years of experience as a community health nursing administrator and taught nursing administration at the master's level. She also administered the Continuing Education Program at the College of Nursing. Her background and work provided a broad perspective on issues that are of critical importance to nurse executives and managers.

Sue Moorhead, PhD, RN, is editor starting with Volume 9. Sue has years of experience in administration as an army nurse and currently is an assistant professor at the University of Iowa. The military provided her with a diverse clinical background and a broad perspective of administrative issues in nursing. She currently teaches undergraduate students at the College of Nursing.

The editorial board consists of faculty teaching in the nursing administration program at Iowa and selected nurse administrators associated with the program. The board meets three to four times a year with the series editor, helps identify the emerging issues and prospective authors, and assists the editor with manuscript review. Iowa's growing program in nursing administration, including study at the doctoral level, makes this an ideal setting to support this publication. A National Advisory Board consisting of nursing administrators, both academic and practicing, advises the editorial board on pertinent topics and authors where needed.

The authors are distinguished nurse administrators, educators, and researchers chosen for their expertise in particular areas. While authors have the freedom to pursue an issue as they choose, each is encouraged to address the state of knowledge, future directions, and the controversial questions surrounding the issue, and to propose one or more options for resolution. Beginning with Volume 7, authors were chosen by a review process following a Call for Abstracts. The Call for Abstracts is mailed and advertised in various journals and newsletters during the months of February through September each year.

The publisher of the series, beginning with Volume 7, is Sage Publications, Inc. Mosby-Year Book, Inc., published Volumes 3 through 6, and Volumes 1 and 2 were published by Addison-Wesley.

All of us involved in this series believe that it will benefit not only those who teach and practice nursing administration but the entire nursing profession and, most important, the patients we serve. We welcome your comments and suggestions.

—Diane Huber, PhD, RN, FAAN
Chairperson, Editorial Board, Volumes 9-10

—Meridean L. Maas, PhD, RN, FAAN
Chairperson, Editorial Board, Volumes 5-8

—Joanne Comi McCloskey, PhD, RN, FAAN
Chairperson, Editorial Board, Volumes 1-4

Introduction

While it is indisputable that nursing is preparing to meet the increased demands for databased outcomes as well as embrace new opportunities for meeting the health needs of its clients, the chasm between the end of the 20th century and the beginning of the 21st century is conspicuous. Major efforts to create adequate information infrastructures within organizations/agencies, systems, and networks are shadowed by demands for national infrastructures that are responsive to international imperatives. At the same time that nurses strive to identify key data and information that capture the process of care and the client response to that care on local, state, and regional levels, immediate national and international standardization imperatives are pressing. All the while nursing is striving to identify clearly its unique contribution to care delivery, the necessity for multidisciplinary and interdisciplinary activities is acute. The collection of chapters in this volume represents a sensitivity to these demands, dichotomies, and possibilities. The volume represents future visions, strategies for acknowledging and accepting the information-oriented paradigm shift, and tips and issues in achieving implementation of information technologies and resources now.

Part I, Visions for Nursing in a New Millennium, highlights three innovations that represent efforts of national, and potentially international, import. Warren and Harris clearly describe the unique as well as shared knowledge requirements for Advanced Practice Nurses (APNs). Further, these authors charge APNs to assume a leadership role in developing an information culture that fosters a united effort to develop new knowledge and skills in nursing. An innovative approach to addressing data needs for the complex decision-making needs of nurse managers and administrators is described by Huber and Delaney. They outline the development process and product of the Nursing

Management Minimum Data Set (NMMDS) and the potential these data have to empower resource and outcome decision making. The pioneering effort to develop and test a virtual nursing collaboratory is described by Goodwin, Turner, Sower, and Yensen. These authors provide a stimulating discussion of trust, autonomy, and energy issues within the framework of doing cooperative work in a new world changed by the information paradigm.

The pioneering innovation focus of Part I is complemented by attention to strategies and skills for nurse administrators who are entering the information age in Part II, Strategies for an Information Revolution. Shellenbarger and Zuraikat present an excellent summary of electronic resources and user-friendly suggestions for applying these tools. Scherb discusses an employee performance evaluation strategy that capitalizes on data and information available within clinical and administrative information systems. Kellum and Tatum discuss innovative interactive computer applications for meeting the clinical, educational, and administrative needs of nursing practice. They focus on the evaluation of specific applications to promote efficient, effective, and productive clinical decision making by nurses. Managers and administrators who are approaching implementation of an information system will find Ireson and Velotta's chapter helpful. Layman, Funk, and Cobb conclude Part II with a specific illustration of the use of the Internet/Web technology to foster research utilization.

The last section of this volume, Tips From the Information Innovators: Creating Change Across Health Care Settings, highlights case studies that describe use of a variety of information technologies across different settings. Behrenbeck, Timm, Gudlin, and Briske's work introduces Part III. They describe the implementation of a comprehensive point-of-care clinical information system in a large tertiary care center and conclude by identifying critical success factors and lessons learned. Brokel, Hawkos, Getman, Schumacher, and Schwichtenberg highlight the challenges of designing unique solutions for coordinating care in an integrated delivery network. Their focus on unique clinical and information systems needs in rural, sparsely populated regions is particular useful. Owens-Vance, Kraft, and Lang provide another picture of implementing a clinical information system across multiple settings within a national health care system for the Veteran's Health Administration electronic patient record.

The remaining authors focus outside the acute care delivery model. McGuire concentrates on care of patients and caregivers within the home. This case study, describing the use of ComputerLink to meet needs of Alzheimer's patients and families in their home, is particularly useful in detailing evaluation of the cost effectiveness of such interventions. Kowalski extends our understanding of the relevancy of Minimum Data Set efforts by describing several case studies that incorporated the Minimum Data Set (MDS) mandated by the Health Care Finance Administration (HCFA); the power of data to advance practice is clear. In the final chapter, the capability of information technologies to impact clinical practice in community settings is aptly addressed by Bargstadt. The capacity of integrated systems to provide access to clinical, financial, and personnel data and information to serve individual clients, groups of clients, and the community as client is clearly described.

Enjoy these shared works. Welcome the opportunity to network with the authors. Also share the vision of a day when each of us, whether clinicians, managers, administrators, researchers, or educators, have the data, information, and knowledge we need to provide expanding creative, responsible, and innovative care.

—Sue Moorhead, PhD, RN
—Connie Delaney, PhD, RN

PART I

Visions for Nursing
in a New Millennium

Three innovations of potentially transnational consequence are presented in this segment. In Chapter 1, Warren and Harris clearly acknowledge the foundation of data, information, and knowledge used by both Advanced Practice Nurses (APNs) and other nurses in practice. Their focus, however, is on articulating strategies that will address the APNs' requisiteness for greater depth and breadth of knowledge, greater synthesis of data, and more complex interventions than nurses use in other practice roles. The authors outline "thrival" strategies that APNs must deploy to meet the challenges and opportunities created by the computer-based patient environment and to survive in the contemporary health care systems. APNs must delineate the knowledge structure of advanced nursing practice; create and develop an information culture where information is perceived as valuable (not perceived as a threat); and unite APNs to develop new knowledge and tools.

Huber and Delaney describe in Chapter 2 a recent innovation, the Nursing Management Minimum Data Set (NMMDS). The development of the NMMDS arose from the acknowledgment of the complex decision making required by nurse managers and administrators in a health care system that is being revolutionized and transformed by the emerging information technologies. This complex decision making requires extensive data and information that captures the context within which care delivery occurs—data and information that go beyond the core clinical data. Clearly, adoption of the NMMDS will provide the infrastructure of data needed to empower nurse managers and administrators to make databased decisions efficiently and effectively, in a more timely manner. Justifying resource expenditures and outcomes realized, managing large interdisciplinary health teams, and determining the added value that nursing brings to health care improvements experienced by clients will result from linking the NMMDS with clinical data and information.

Goodwin, Turner, Sower, and Yensen describe an extraordinary pioneering effort toward a fundamentally new way of effecting both nursing administration and nursing science in the 21st century in Chapter 3. Development of a Virtual Nursing Information Collaboratory provides an opportunity for nurse administrators from around the world to communicate and collaborate in administrative problem solving, strategic planning, and outcome research. These authors describe the collaboratory concept; the development, testing, and pilot projects of a specific collaboratory model (Virtual Nursing Administration Collaboratory for Patient Outcomes Research); and provide an excellent synthesis of the development issues arising from this cooperative work that will create a new paradigm. Of particular note is the authors' consideration of such factors as trust within social systems, autonomy issues, and sustaining energy and momentum for this innovative work.

CHAPTER 1

Challenges and Opportunities for Advanced Practice Nurses in a Computer-Based Patient Record Environment

Judith J. Warren
Marcelline R. Harris

Advanced practice nurses (APNs) share the foundation of data, information, and knowledge used in basic nursing practice. The difference for the APN is that there are clear expectations that the depth and breadth of knowledge are greater, the synthesis of data is greater, and skills and interventions are more complex. This chapter addresses the expectations of the APN and opportunities for synthesizing data and developing knowledge applications for nursing within the computer-based patient record environment. Three "thrival" strategies are clearly described, including delineating the knowledge structure of nursing practice, creating and developing an information culture, and uniting APNs to develop knowledge tools. Clearly, APNs must possess the sophisticated clinical and organizational knowledge required for the identification of data needed to document nursing practice, design interfaces between nurses and the computer that work, and design clinical databases.

In attempting to arrive at the truth, I have applied everywhere for information, but in scarcely an instance have I been able to obtain hospital records fit for any purpose of comparison. If they could be obtained they would enable us to decide many other questions besides the one alluded

3

to. They would show the subscribers how their money was being spent, what good was really being done with it, or whether the money was not doing mischief rather than good.

Nightingale, *Notes on Hospitals,* 1863

More than a century after Nightingale bemoaned the lack of information to answer key questions about health care and its effects on patients, advanced practice nurses (APNs) still find themselves "applying everywhere for information." Using data to structure information and contribute to knowledge building is as much a challenge to contemporary APNs as it was to Nightingale. Despite this, many recognize APNs as important participants in changing systems of care delivery and support the increased use of APNs (Institute of Medicine, 1996).

The participation of APNs in contemporary health care systems is based on APNs' implicit foundation as "knowledge workers." The knowledge the APN brings to health care, whether as a clinician, consultant, in education, as a researcher, or in a manager role option, is attributable to the specific educational preparation and unique employment positions that enable the APN to interact and communicate with all players involved in delivering health care. APNs are prepared, by virtue of their graduate education in nursing, with (a) critical analysis skills required to identify, collect, and interpret complex clinical and organizational data; (b) systematic problem-solving skills to support change; (c) advanced and specialized knowledge about specific clinical populations and health care systems; and (d) theory-derived and research-based knowledge to support care. The employment positions of APNs require communication and interaction with patients and families along the continuum of care, a wide spectrum of providers based in diverse settings, complex systems that control access and payment, and vendors that market products to support interaction and communication. The APN is uniquely prepared and positioned to address the data, information, and knowledge relationships described by Graves and Corcoran (1989).

APNs are now explicitly challenged to use this preparation and position within changing health care systems that are increasingly reliant on electronic methods for data, information, and knowledge. Fortunately, APN knowledge is convergent with the broad informatics requirements of health care. There is a need to identify and obtain patient, management, and environmental *data* used to generate *information* that accurately reflects the reality of practice and supports clinical, organizational, and health care system decision making. This information enables APNs and others to create new *knowledge* for and about the health care management of individuals and populations within complex organizations and across integrated care delivery systems. Equally important is the development of new knowledge as a basis for the preparation of the next generation of APNs and other health care workers. Reflecting on the role of APNs after health care reform, Donley (1995) wrote, "Nurses have assumed the management of the health care team by design or default. . . . It is an exciting and creative time to be in advanced practice" (p. 88). The computer-based patient record environment presents an exciting and important venue in which the APN can creatively and uniquely contribute to data, information, and knowledge needs that are prerequisite to deciding many other questions besides the one alluded to. APNs would show the subscribers how their money was being spent, what good was really being done with it, or whether the money was not doing mischief rather than good (to paraphrase Nightingale).

THE CPR ENVIRONMENT

The computer-based patient record (CPR) environment is characterized as a very complex, evolving, and highly political component of the health care industry (Dick & Steen, 1991; Henry, 1995b; Zielstorff, Hudgings, & Grobe, 1993). There are expectations, and some evidence, that computerization of health care information provides a method for improving health care and reducing its cost. Automating the current paper-based patient record or creating very large databases, similar to those used by government and industry, will not accomplish this. Discipline-specific knowledge engineers, vendors, and others representing the entire health care team are working collaboratively to develop new ways of looking at patient and health care data. The Computer-based Patient Record Institute (CPRI), through the use of experts, is facilitating a fundamental change in information gathering, use, and access (CPRI, 1993). The CPR and the computer-based patient record system (CPRS), as defined by the CPRI, are the foundation of a new view of the health care information system (CPRI, 1995).

The infrastructure within the CPR has three essential elements required to support quality nursing care of patients and families (Henry, Holzemer, Tallberg, & Grobe, 1995). The first element is a set of standardized nursing vocabularies that describe patient problems and characteristics, nursing interventions, patient outcomes sensitive to the effects of nursing care (Zielstorff, 1995), the intensity of patient care, and the resources required to provide care. The second element is a set of computer-based methods to examine linkages between and among the variables listed in the first element and to analyze variations in nursing practice (Holzemer & Reilly, 1995). These methods must be risk adjusted and must reveal the relationships between the processes and outcomes of care. The last element is an integrated clinical information management environment that collects and reports data to the clinician during patient care. This feedback on performance and patient response to the clinician is essential for quality nursing care. In fact, these three elements are essential for all health care disciplines. A multidisciplinary initiative is essential to the work of developing the CPR environment.

Other factors are also influencing the CPR environment. First, the minicomputer and microcomputer technology has revolutionized the concept of data processing and accessing. Computer workstations are powerful, convenient, and small enough to be placed in patient care areas, even at the bedside; in the examination room; and in the patient's home. Second, the entertainment and communications industry, with its focus on improving interactive games and virtual reality experiences, creating the special effects for television and motion picture films, and bringing interactive communication technology to the home, has pushed the vision of the role of computers in data and information management. Third, nursing (in fact, all health care disciplines) needs an integrated CPR environment to maximize the benefits to the health care system, minimize cost, maximize opportunities for improving quality patient care, facilitate continuity of care, ensure consistent privacy and security controls, and minimize duplication of data collection and entry for patients and providers (Henry et al., 1995). Finally, given the fact that there will always be a need for humans to interpret computer-processed data and information (Graves & Corcoran, 1989), what opportunities does the CPR environment create for APNs' "thrival" (the ability to find new opportunities to thrive and succeed; Chenevert, 1985) in the CPR environment?

"THRIVAL" STRATEGIES FOR THE APN

There are strategies APNs can deploy to meet the challenges and the opportunities created by the CPR environment. These strategies include the development and use of standardized data elements to delineate the knowledge structure of nursing practice; communication and collaboration in creating and developing a multidisciplinary health care information culture; and unification with other APNs, building on the perspective of specialty roles, to develop new knowledge tools and data-driven patient care and organization solutions.

Delineate the Knowledge Structure of Nursing Practice

Zielstorff et al. (1993) state that nursing needs

> knowledgeable nurses who view data and information in clinical practice as essential for care management, care improvement, and nursing knowledge development. Such a dynamic view implies that nurses clearly understand what data are important, how these data might best be used for differing purposes, and that using them benefits nurses. (p. 41)

This statement is based on the assumption that nurses have the knowledge, skills, and abilities to work with data and have the motivation to engage in this work. The structure of nursing knowledge is based on *Nursing's Social Policy Statement* (American Nurses Association [ANA], 1995), *Standards of Clinical Nursing Practice* (American Nurses Association [ANA], 1991), standards of specialty nursing organizations, clinical guideline development (Field & Lohr, 1992; Marek, 1995; McCormick, Moore, & Siegel, 1994), policies and procedures of the organization, nursing care standards of the organization, and nursing research. The essential question to be answered is: What data are both of interest uniquely to nursing and shared with other disciplines? The APN needs to understand the knowledge structure of nursing—how the art and science of nursing is arranged and its relationships—to ensure that the appropriate data and information are included in the CPR and CPRS.

Standardized vocabularies have developed so that patient record information can be aggregated to meet the needs identified by Nightingale and today's nurse leaders (Lang, 1995). "Not only are standardized vocabularies needed to clarify meanings and communication between providers, but codes are needed in computer databases in order to store and retrieve data. Computers are not able to find meaning in text material" (Warren, Delaney, & Ryan, 1997, p. 390). Codes are numbers, letters, or both, that are used to represent abstract concepts such as nursing vocabularies. These codes can be stored, retrieved, and reassembled into a text representation of the data. These characteristics of codes are why databases can be queried and why appropriate representation of concepts is essential.

Reasons supporting the use of standardized vocabularies within nursing are not widely understood, and in fact, resistance to using standardized vocabularies is evident. A work group at a nursing informatics conference answered the question with the following: to describe consistently what nurses do, define the body of nursing knowledge, ensure clarity of meaning, permit comparability of practice and cost, reduce cost of information systems technology, reduce staff training costs and errors of practice, and improve the quality of multidisciplinary coordination of care. A second work group identified issues for staff nurses: Standardized vocabularies must resemble the language they use, be tested, map to staff's common language, and map to synonyms (Henry et al., 1995). Warren (1997) noted that "a standardized vocabulary facilitates the abstraction, summarization, and aggregation of unique, individual patient data into meaningful patterns and themes so that accurate communication of information about the patient can occur between providers and administrators" (p. 390). By supporting the use of standardized nursing vocabularies, APNs can assist with documentation while enhancing the expression and development of nursing knowledge.

Not only are coded, standardized vocabularies needed in an information-driven world, but recognized data sets (see Table 1.1 for examples) are needed so that institutions may communicate with their internal and external worlds. These data sets specify the data elements (e.g., nursing diagnoses, nursing interventions, unique nurse identifier, or hours of care—a calculated variable) and how those elements are to be recorded or calculated. The first data set to be developed and, subsequently, recognized by the ANA is the Nursing Minimum Data Set (Werley & Lang, 1988). The second data set to be developed in nursing is the Nursing Management Minimum Data Set (Huber & Delaney, in press). This data set was developed under the auspices of the American Organization of Nurse Executives and will be submitted to the ANA for recognition after field testing. The American Nurses Association (ANA) has also recognized standardized nursing classification systems that have been incorporated in the meta-thesaurus of the National Library of Medicine (Lang, 1995).

The identification of data elements needed to design electronic clinical databases, document nursing practice, and support human interface with the computer requires sophisticated clinical and organizational knowledge that APNs possess. "Clinical data represent an under-utilized resource, one with great potential to improve patient care delivery. The under-use of data may result partially from the current inability to manage large volumes of data to determine patterns that will be useful for prediction" (Zielstorff et al., 1993, p. 6). A model of a pyramid that represents patient data that is collected once and used many times has been developed by Zielstorff and colleagues (1993). There are five levels in the pyramid: the patient level, the agency level, the community or regional level, the national level, and the global level. Data may be abstracted, summarized, and aggregated at each level and used by a variety of users with different information needs and scope of interest at each level. APNs must be cognizant of these levels so that information, as it is passed on,

TABLE 1.1   Coded, Standardized Vocabularies

Nursing coding schemes and standardized vocabularies
    ANA recognized classifications: NANDA, Nursing Intervention Classification, Omaha
      VNA system, Home Health Care System
    Nursing classification schemes under development: Nursing Outcomes Classification,
      Ozbolt Nursing Vocabulary, Nursing Intervention Lexical Terminology

International Council of Nursing: International Classification of Nursing Process (ICNP)

Related coding schemes of importance to nursing:
    Unified Medical Language System (National Library of Medicine)
    Major coding schemes: ICD-9-CM, CPT-IV, SNOMED International, *DSM-IV*,
      Medicare's Diagnosis Related Groups (DRGs)

---

is useful and accurate for the needs of each level. Health care reform requires more information sharing and reporting than has ever existed in history.

Create and Develop an Information Culture

Communication and collaboration on the development and use of the CPR and CPRS are required within and outside the organization employing APNs to support a culture in which information is perceived as a value, not a threat. To support this within the organization, APNs need to develop alignments with chief information officers, hospital administrators and managers, financial and medical records departments, marketing and public relations offices, medical staff, and other health care disciplines. This not only enhances APNs' understanding about the organization and available resources, but often provides others in the organization with the clinical perspective they need to do their own jobs more effectively. It is much easier to talk and work with familiar people who know and trust a specific APN and his or her skills and abilities.

Bolman and Deal (1991) described an organization's culture as "the pattern of beliefs, values, practices, and artifacts that define for its members who they are and how they do things" (p. 250). The CPR and CPRS introduce dramatically new ways of doing the work of the health care organization, and new job expectations to support that work. This contributes to the renewal and re-creation of the culture, whether or not a change in culture was planned. Connor (1995) viewed the same phenomenon from the perspective of leading during times of rapid change, change so rapid that most individuals and organizations find it difficult to survive. However, rapid change also presents an opportunity to redefine the culture of the organization, "an opportunity for a fundamental shift in how we humans define ourselves, where we are going, and how we will accomplish our goals" (Connor, 1995, p. 4). APNs can make a difference in the culture and the future of the organization and nursing within the organization by providing leadership and use of successful change management strategies.

Under conditions of culture change, organizations and their members will create and use symbols, metaphors, and data to bring meaning out of chaos; clarity to communication; and predictability from uncertainty (Bolman & Deal, 1991). This is the most profound change for an organization's culture to undergo. APNs need to understand that access to data and information creates an open environment where the secrets, myths, and rituals of organizations can no longer be hidden. APNs have the opportunity to help create these symbols, metaphors, and data and, by that, influence the culture of their organizations. Furthermore, APNs are positioned to help the organization to understand and embrace this phenomenon of the CPR environment and the information age.

To support communication and collaboration outside the employing organization, the APN can become involved with different national organizations involved in activities such as standards setting, health care policy and regulation, and professional organizations. Many opportunities exist for involvement (see Table 1.2). APNs, by becoming active in one or more of these organizations or monitoring their work, can ensure that their organization is choosing data and information strategies that will enable them to compete and thrive in a data-driven world. From a broader perspective, APNs can collaborate with others to ensure a nursing voice in the development of standards, policy, and regulation at local, national, and international levels.

APNs, through collaboration and communication, can be leaders who influence the development of a culture that embraces information technology. The CPR environment provides an opportunity for transforming this vision into reality.

Unite APNs to Develop New Knowledge Tools

While the paradigm defining newer systems of care focuses on teamwork, collaboration, and partnerships (Ashkenas, Ulrich, Jick, & Kerr, 1995; Bolman & Deal, 1991; Senge, 1990), specific disciplines and providers are expected to provide evidence, supported by data, that shows the unique effects of their work on outcomes. APNs are challenged to provide meaningful clinical information, as well as information on the contributions APNs make to patient, organizational, and system outcomes (Henry, 1995a). Nursing is not unfamiliar with discussions about the compelling reasons to speak with a unified voice to ensure a nursing presence in health care. However, this discussion takes on new dimensions for the APN in the CPR environment. One reason to present a

TABLE 1.2   Major Organizations Involved in Heath Care Information Standards
           and Policy

Standard-Setting Organizations	Health Care Policy and Regulation	Organizations for Health Care Professionals
Computer-based Patient Record Institute (CPRI)	Agency for Health Care Policy and Research (AHCPR)	American Nurses Association (ANA)
Health Level 7 (HL7)	National Committee on Vital and Health Statistics (NCVHS)	American Organization of Nurse Executives (AONE)
American National Standards Institute-Health Information Standards Board (ANSI-HISB)	Health Care Financing Administration (HCFA)	Center for Healthcare Information Management (AHIMA)
American Society for Testing and Materials (ASTM)	Joint Commission for the Accreditation of Healthcare Organizations (JCAHO)	College of Healthcare Information Management Executives (CHIME)
		Healthcare Information and Management Systems Society (HIMSS)
		American Hospital Association Work Group on the Computer-Based Patient Record
		American Medical Informatics Association (AMIA)

unified APN perspective is that the CPR is being developed for an integrated, computer-based *patient* record system. It is not being developed to support disciplines or specialties within specific disciplines. Only data that provide relevant information to support patient care have a legitimate claim to being present in the CPR.

APNs can unite to develop a strong CPR environment for the patient and also for nursing and other disciplines, instead of engaging in "parallel play" to meet their own data and information needs. This latter approach will only fragment and weaken advanced practice nursing and health care delivery. APNs will require systems that are flexible and able to be modified as data needs change. APNs, using a unified voice to support the information needs of clinicians, administrators, educators, and researchers, are more likely to influence effectively the inclusion of nursing-sensitive data.

A new APN role, the informatics nurse specialist, can facilitate this. The theory of nursing informatics is concerned with the ways nurses use data, information, and knowledge to make decisions about patient care and its delivery (American Nurses Association [ANA], 1994a, 1994b). Furthermore, informatics nurse specialists work with the technologies for information management and processing and how these technologies affect and are affected by the practice of nursing (ANA, 1994a). The American Nurses Association defines this new specialty as the one "that integrates nursing science, computer science, and information science in identifying, collecting, processing, and managing data and information to support nursing practice, administration, education, research, and the expansion of nursing knowledge" (ANA, 1994a, p. 3).

However, other APN roles also need to develop competency in the analysis and evaluation of data and information requirements for nursing practice. An example of this competency would be to understand the implications of the structure of a clinical database. The structure of a clinical database enables data linkages and the determination of variations in cost (Henry et al., 1995). All APNs need to become aware of possible influences and implications of information technology, such as clinical decision support and practice reminders, workstation designs, data acquisition/entry and data retrieval methods, data integrity and reliability, and patient information confidentiality. ANAs' computer design criteria should be used by APNs participating in the selection and purchase of computer hardware and software that will support nursing data needs and the needs of others (Zielstorff, McHugh, & Clinton, 1988). Currently, major health care computer and software vendors are partnering with niche vendors who have systems for laboratory, physiologic critical care data, patient acuity, and so forth, to improve their market share. Essential questions such as where the data have been, how they were transformed or manipulated, how they were stored or lost from the database, whether the data are automatically placed in all relevant tables or must be reentered, and how easy it will be and how long it will take to retrieve data from the database, are shared across APN functions.

CONCLUSION

APNs will thrive in the CPR environment if they carry out strategies that not only strengthen their own role as knowledge workers, but also contribute to the information needs of others within health care. APNs are challenged to recognize their implicit strength as knowledge workers and to turn this strength into opportunities explicitly to demonstrate their critical role in designing effective, efficient health care. The knowledge structures that support and reveal quality patient care must be developed. APNs possess the sophisticated clinical and organization knowledge required for the identification of data elements needed to document nursing practice, design of the nurse's interface with the computer, and design of the clinical database. The final winning strategy is being involved in developing, implementing, and evaluating the CPR and the CPRS at their institutions.

REFERENCES

American Nurses Association. (1991). *The standards of clinical nursing practice.* Washington, DC: Author.

American Nurses Association. (1994a). *The scope of practice for nursing informatics.* Washington, DC: Author.

American Nurses Association. (1994b). *The standards of practice for nursing informatics.* Washington, DC: Author.

American Nurses Association. (1995). *Nursing's social policy statement.* Washington, DC: Author.

Ashkenas, R., Ulrich, D., Jick, T., & Kerr, S. (1995). *The boundaryless organization: Breaking the chains of organizational structure.* San Francisco: Jossey-Bass.

Bolman, L. G., & Deal, T. G. (1991). *Reframing organizations.* San Francisco: Jossey-Bass.

Chenevert, M. (1985). *Pro-nurse handbook: Designed for the nurse who wants to thrive professionally.* St. Louis, MO: C. V. Mosby.

Connor, D. R. (1995). *Managing at the speed of change: How resilient managers succeed and prosper where others fail.* New York: Villiard.

CPRI. (1993). *Position paper: Computer-based patient record standards.* Chicago: Computer-based Patient Record Institute.

CPRI. (1995). *CPR and CPRS definitions.* Chicago: Computer-based Patient Record Institute.

Dick, R. S., & Steen, E. B. (1991). *The computer-based patient record: An essential technology for health care.* Washington, DC: National Academy Press.

Donley, Sr. R. (1995). Advanced practice nursing after health care reform. *Nursing Economics, 13*(2), 84-88.

Field, M. J., & Lohr, K. N. (Eds.). (1992). *Guidelines for clinical practice: From development to use.* Washington, DC: National Academy Press.

Graves, J. R., & Corcoran, S. (1989). The study of nursing informatics. *Image: Journal of Nursing Scholarship, 21,* 227-233.

Henry, S. B. (1995a). Informatics: Essential infrastructure for quality assessment and improvement in nursing. *Journal of the American Medical Informatics Association, 2*(3), 169-182.

Henry, S. B. (1995b). Nursing informatics: State of the science. *Journal of Advanced Nursing, 22,* 1182-1192.

Henry, S. B., Holzemer, W. L., Tallberg, M., & Grobe, S. J. (1995). *Informatics: The infrastructure for quality assessment and improvement in nursing.* San Francisco: UC Nursing Press.

Holzemer, W. L., & Reilly, C. A. (1995). Variables, variability, and variations research: Implications for medical informatics. *Journal of the American Medical Informatics Association, 2,* 183-190.

Huber, D., & Delaney, C. (in press). *The Nursing Management Minimum Data Set (NMMDS) for nurse executives project.* Chicago: American Organization of Nurse Executives.

Institute of Medicine. (1996). *Nursing staff in hospitals and nursing homes.* Washington, DC: National Academy Press.

Lang, N. M. (Ed.). (1995). *Nursing data systems: The emerging framework.* Washington, DC: American Nurses Association.

Marek, K. D. (1995). *Manual to develop guidelines.* Washington, DC: American Nurses Association.

McCormick, K. A., Moore, S. R., & Siegel, R. A. (1994). *Clinical practice guideline development: Methodology perspectives* (AHCPR Pub. No. 95-0009). Washington, DC: U.S. Department of Health and Human Services.

Nightingale, F. (1863). *Notes on hospitals.* London: Longman, Green, Longman, Roberts, and Green.

Senge, P. M. (1990). *The fifth discipline: The art and practice of the learning organization.* Garden City, NY: Doubleday Currency.

Warren, J. J., Delaney, C., & Ryan, P. (1997). Health care reform in an electronic world. In M. J. Rantz & P. LeMone (Eds.), *Classification of nursing diagnoses: Proceedings of the Twelfth Conference of the North American Nursing Diagnosis Association* (pp. 385-399). Glendale, CA: CINAHL Information Systems.

Werley, H. H., & Lang, N. M. (Eds.). (1988). *Identification of the Nursing Minimum Data Set.* New York: Springer.

Zielstorff, R. D. (1995). Capturing and using clinical outcome data: Implications for information systems design. *Journal of the American Medical Informatics Association, 2,* 191-196.

Zielstorff, R. D., Hudgings, C. I., & Grobe, S. J. (1993). *Next-generation nursing information systems: Essential characteristics for professional practice.* Washington, DC: American Nurses Association.

Zielstorff, R. D., McHugh, M. L., & Clinton, J. (1988). *Computer design criteria for systems that support the nursing process.* Kansas City, MO: American Nurses Association.

CHAPTER 2

Nursing Management Data for Nursing Information Systems

Diane Huber
Connie Delaney

The Nursing Management Minimum Data Set (NMMDS) addresses the need for core data to support nursing management decisions. The NMMDS is a useful adjunct to a clinical computerized information system incorporating standardized language to capture clinical patient/client data. This chapter features the NMMDS and its relationship to a nursing management information system development cycle, nursing management practice, and related standardized performance "report cards." For nurses to acquire greater professional effectiveness, both clinical and management data need to be computerized and available for coordination and integration decisions within a multidisciplinary care environment.

The 21st century is projected to bring a patient/client focus for health care in general and to the practice of nursing specifically. It is anticipated that patients will transition among seamless settings, cared for by an increasingly interdisciplinary care delivery team, which will result in less emphasis on

AUTHORS' NOTE: The authors wish to acknowledge the contributions of Peg Mehmert, Janet Specht, Phyllis Schultz, Heidi Nobiling, Sally Bachman, Marilyn Bedell, Donna Fosbinder, and Karen Bossard; Advisory Board members: Marjorie Beyers, June Clark, Leah Curtin, JoEllen Koerner, Norma Lang, Judith Ryan, Walter Sermeus, Franklin Shaffer, Roy Simpson, and Joyce Verran; and consultants: Kitty Buckwalter, Gloria Bulechek, Geraldene Felton, Marion Johnson, Kathy Kelly, Meridean Maas, Joanne McCloskey, Toni Tripp-Reimer, and Frank Kohout. We are grateful to them.

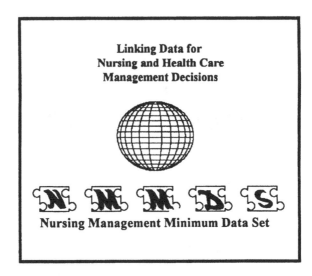

Figure 2.1. Linking Data
SOURCE: Copyright © D. Huber and C. Delaney. Reprinted with permission.

the individual provider. The complex decision making that will be essential to this new paradigm will require the availability of management data that cross settings and are available more quickly than is possible with manual retrieval. Databased decisions cannot be made rapidly enough with manually generated data in current and future dynamic environments (Maas & Mulford, 1989).

The information society's evolutionary development out of an industrial society has been chronicled for years. The innovation of the silicon chip advanced the processing and communication of information farther than futurists could have predicted only a few years ago. Gates (1995) predicted that people's daily lives would be revolutionized and transformed by the emerging technologies. Health care, too, will be affected by the changes already evident in the half-life of new technology.

TECHNOLOGY AND THE NURSING PROFESSION

The nursing profession is recognizing and acknowledging the significant trends that are being fostered by technological advances. Nurses are learning to use technological tools to benefit patients/clients and nurses in the delivery of nursing and health care. Studies have suggested that time savings in indirect nursing activities and more complete charting are positive outcomes of clinical information systems (Axford & Carter, 1996). Similar benefits are now being proposed and need to be demonstrated for nursing management information systems.

Nurse managers make complex decisions about care management, including forecasting and predicting scenarios. They need data and information to make the best decisions rapidly in an uncertain and risky environment. This chapter profiles the Nursing Management Minimum Data Set (NMMDS) as the research-based standardized nursing management data set that can be used to form the core components of a management information system for nurses and nurse managers. The NMMDS provides the infrastructure of data nurse managers need to perform their job responsibilities effectively, make timely complex decisions in practice, and manage the large interdisciplinary teams contributing to care delivery.

INFORMATION INFRASTRUCTURE

The use of information technology means more than nurses learning to use computers. While that may be a necessary first step, nurses have much to gain by participating in the engineering of nursing information systems that expedite information management and processing. This is because, fundamentally, information is a resource to be managed and a source of power to achieve goals. Nurses face the challenge of acquiring methods and skills in controlling and linking information and thereby harnessing the potential of integrated information management for strategic planning and daily management.

Some non-nursing examples of improvements in patient/client care information handling include the use of "smart cards" that contain a health history, billing information, other vital health information, or combinations of these. These wallet-sized cards can be used to streamline admission, chart control, billing, and record keeping. Telemedicine and telenursing strategies can be used for diagnosis and treatment, as well as education for greater health awareness. Hospital documentation strategies are moving into sophisticated systems where physician-dictated notes are represented by an icon until transcribed. Clicking on the icon results in playing an audio recording of the dictation.

Nursing, too, has responded to the information age. Numerous nursing-related technological and informatics innovations have been developed and implemented. For example, nursing leaders have identified the critical elements of a Nursing Minimum Data Set (NMDS; Werley & Lang, 1988). Nursing leaders have developed several standardized classifications to define nursing practice, such as the North American Nursing Diagnosis Association's (NANDA) classification (North American Nursing Diagnosis Association,

[NANDA], 1994); Nursing Interventions Classification (NIC; Iowa Intervention Project, 1996); Nursing-Sensitive Outcomes Classification (NOC; Maas,
Johnson, & Kraus, 1996); the Omaha System (Martin & Scheet, 1992); and
Saba's Classification (Saba, 1992). Professional organizations have supported
the need for nursing information for clinical practice, research, and administration, such as the American Nurses Association's Next Generation Nursing
Information Systems resource (Zielstorff, Hudgings, & Grobe, 1993); Information Research Priorities (National Center for Nursing Research [NCNR],
1992); and the American Organization of Nurse Executives' support of the need
for management data collection and analysis development. The question is how
soon will nurses be able to track, monitor, query, and display analyses of
nursing care activities, time spent, costs, variances, and quality data on demand
and in real time?

Nursing is somewhat behind in the development of nursing care and nursing
management information systems because, until recently, the necessary infrastructure of standardized language that is essential in order to program information systems was not fully developed or accepted. Moreover, because nursing has been at the core of all patient/client care delivery and support, all
nursing applications are dependent on the development of these ancillary
systems first. Fundamentally, nurses need to analyze their care activities and
what else supports care, then determine what data need to be collected. Standardized definitions and measures need to be developed and consensus agreement derived for all data deemed necessary. When nurses identify what data to
collect, computerized systems can be developed to manage and process the data
into information that is usable by nurses or nurse managers to make decisions
in the integration, coordination, management, and delivery of nursing services.
The appropriate data infrastructure provides nurses with the discipline-
specific information needed to make decisions and develop persuasive fact-
based arguments for improving care. Otherwise, decisions are made on in-
stinct, tradition, or intuition—and anecdotes form the database.

Recent attempts to influence public policy have demonstrated that persuasive strategies need to be based on data, not anecdotes. This was clearly
demonstrated in the 1995 Institute of Medicine (IOM) hearings and is reflected
in the 1995 Pew Report (Pew Health Professions Commission, 1995). The
recent IOM report on nurse staffing (Wunderlich, Sloan, & Davis, 1996)
highlighted the need for standardized variables relating to the quality of care
in hospitals: "One of the research challenges in determining the relationship
between staffing and quality of care has been the difficulty of isolating the
factors (and the relative importance of these factors) that are involved in
producing improved patient outcomes" (p. 9). The IOM committee noted a

national "lack of systematic and ongoing monitoring and evaluating of the effects of organizational redesign and reconfiguration of staffing on patient outcomes" (Wunderlich et al., 1996, p. 9). The Pew Report observed that

> Clearly, the new system will be driven by information. The communications and information technologies that have emerged over the past decade have become important drivers of the emerging health care system. Without such resources the integration and management of care at the levels currently anticipated would simply not be possible. To remain a vital part of a complex, managed, information-driven system health professions must be able to manage and use large volumes of scientific, technological and patient information in a way that helps them deliver effective clinical care in the context of community and system needs. (Pew Health Professions Commission, 1995, p. 6)

The Joint Commission on Accreditation of Healthcare Organizations (JCAHO; 1994) recognized the importance of the management of information by including in its *1995 Accreditation Manual for Hospitals* a set of standards for information management planning. Standard IM.3 is, "When feasible, uniform data definitions and methods for capturing data are in place" (JCAHO, 1994, p. 55). Standard IM.8 is, "The information-management function provides for the definition, capture, analysis, transmission, and reporting of data and information that can be aggregated to support managerial decisions and operations, performance-improvement activities, and patient care" (JCAHO, 1994, p. 60). Standard IM.10 specifically addresses the use of comparative performance data and information, using external reference databases for comparative purposes.

An effectively designed and managed computerized information system can augment and improve nursing management decision making and subsequently impact the success of the institution (Anderson, Dobal, & Blessing, 1992). The NMMDS is the critical core set of nursing management data needed to meet the pressing need for management information in nursing practice. The NMMDS fits easily into the development cycle of a nursing information system.

DEVELOPMENT CYCLE

Managed care initiatives, competition, and capitation-based reimbursement systems have increasingly fueled an interest in information systems as a way to follow and manage the consumption of scarce resources in health care systems. Systems of reimbursement in health care that place providers at risk for the quantity and quality of care delivered have highlighted the deficiencies of data collection and usage (Ross, 1986). Targeted data elements specific to competitive contracting initiatives appear to be essential for organizational survival in a capitated, managed care payment system. Thus organizations have begun to focus resources on developing outcomes measurements and sophisticated cost identification analyses. In this same manner, nurses have a renewed opportunity to examine the cost and quality aspects of nursing care. The environment is primed for nursing to move forward in developing, refining, and linking essential databases that encompass crucial nursing-sensitive elements. Nurses must first identify nursing data needs; then they will be able to use the subsequent information to contribute to interdisciplinary care delivery efforts and to negotiate for needed scarce resources.

In the past, nurses were responsible for collecting, handling, documenting, and coordinating large volumes of information in health care systems (Zielstorff, McHugh, & Clinton, 1988). Even as far back as the 1960s, it was estimated that as much as 40% of nurses' time was spent managing and communicating information (Jydstrup & Gross, 1966; Richart, 1970; Zielstorff et al., 1988). Today, nurses need to know exactly how their time is spent and what information they are managing in order to manage complexity while being effective and productively efficient. Accountability and competitiveness depend on accurate and reliable information processing.

The development cycle for a nursing management information system starts with activity analysis and data elements identification and ends with linkage to other relational databases. Figure 2.2 displays the system development cycle for nursing management data. This model draws on the contemporary multiview of developing systems that emphasizes the relationship between the care environment and the organization (Tan, 1995). Nurses first need to analyze management activities and information needs for management decisions. This includes not only identifying what information is needed to address which practice/management questions or goals, but also who makes the decision and what the decision-making process is. From this analysis, nurses can identify the data that are important. Knowing what data to collect means the identification of the core, essential data elements or variables needed to capture the data that must be available in order to answer important questions about the management of care and care delivery.

Each element can then be defined. Only with an accepted, standardized definition will data comparison across sites and settings of care be possible. Clarity of definition is a critical consideration for nurses to be accurate in understanding and applying the definition in practice.

Step 5 is to develop a standardized measure for each element. In research terms, the measure is the operational definition. The capture of the data becomes a reality by means of employing the measure to quantify the data and

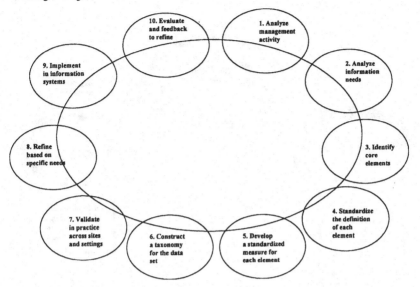

Figure 2.2. Nursing Management Information System Development Cycle

encode it in the information system. The integrity of the data reflect the precision and sensitivity of the measurement of the data element. A taxonomy can then be constructed in Step 6.

Steps 7 and 8 involve validation of the care elements and their measures in practice and further refinement. All data sets need to incorporate continual growth and refinement as new knowledge becomes available and as practice environments evolve.

The 9th step in a nursing management information system's development cycle is actual implementation or adoption of the data set. The cycle continues (Step 10) with evaluation and feedback to continually refine the nursing management information system. Evaluation data feed back into the beginning of the cycle as a continuous process.

Throughout the developmental cycle, attention to the linkage possibilities to other management data sets such as organizational financial or personnel data sets and clinical data sets is paramount. Part of the power of the NMMDS resides in the possibility of linking clinical and management information in order to more robustly capture data that can be used to analyze care and service outcomes. Figure 2.3 depicts this linkage.

THE NMMDS

Evaluating and using data effectively is an essential part of a nurse's expertise. However, without nursing-identified core data being captured in information

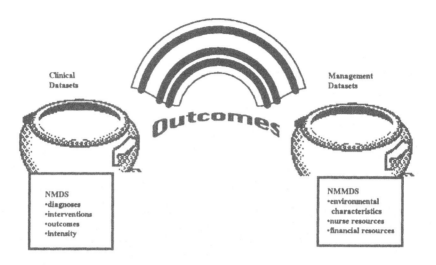

Figure 2.3. Linkage of Clinical and Management Data Sets

systems, nursing's value is invisible, others claim credit for nursing's accomplishments, or both. With efforts under way to identify and define clinical information systems, the lack of nursing management data sets became apparent. The NMMDS research project was undertaken to address this gap.

Evidence exists for the need for an NMMDS. The Priority Expert Panel on Nursing Informatics of the National Center for Nursing Research (NCNR, 1992) identified in Research Program Goal #2 the need to develop methods to build databases of clinical information and of management information (including staffing, charge capture, turnover, and vacancy rates) and to analyze relationships among them. Simpson (1993) noted that the lack of a nationally accepted NMMDS stands in the way of nurses' influencing national health policy. Recognizing this, the American Organization of Nurse Executives' (AONE) Board of Directors set the establishment and acceptance of a uniform NMMDS as a top priority in their 1993 Strategic Activities. A resolution at the 1996 American Nurses Association's House of Delegates called for the advancement of the NMMDS; a similar resolution was passed at the 1996 Iowa Nurses Association annual convention.

Morrison and Keyes (1989) researched the nursing management literature to seek comprehensive and uniform management elements. They were unsuccessful. The NMMDS coprincipal investigators (co-PIs) found the same void. As a result, Huber and Delaney formed a research team to identify and develop a research-based NMMDS. They assembled members with expertise in uniform data sets, nursing management across a variety of settings, and nursing informatics. The result of the early work was a list of 18 elements and definitions (Huber, Delaney, Crossley, Mehmert, & Ellerbe, 1992). This initial work also assessed the clarity, necessity, and collectability of the core NMMDS elements in acute care and resulted in a consensus on the data elements needed by nurse executives in acute care hospital-based practice.

Following the development of consensus in acute care practice, the researchers investigated and compared the validity and usefulness of the NMMDS in nonacute care settings, including long-term care, ambulatory care, occupational health, and home health/community health settings. The research used several methods: expert opinions, consensus surveys, and a consensus-building invitational workshop. Expert nurse opinions were solicited, and surveys were sent to nurses in selected nonhospital settings to determine the adaptability of the core elements to each setting. It became evident that further consensus-related activities were necessary concerning definitional and measurement issues. The invitational workshop, held in January 1996, brought nursing experts together with the research team to refine the data set. The workshop, sponsored by the American Organization of Nurse Executives, developed a cross-settings refinement of 17 basic NMMDS elements applicable to all settings (see Figure 2.4) with standardized definitions and measures (Delaney & Huber, 1996).

ELEMENTS OF THE NMMDS

The 17 elements of the NMMDS are divided into three main categories: the environment, nurse resources, and financial resources. The major activities of nurse managers are reflected in these three domains.

The *environment* domain includes nine variables that provide a profile of the environment that is coordinated by the nurse manager at the unit or service level. The unit or service level is defined as a center of excellence, a service program, a cluster by level of care, or may be called service/product line (Delaney & Huber, 1996). The context within which nursing services are provided to patients/clients is encompassed by these nine elements. It is important to describe precisely the type of nursing delivery unit/service center; population(s) served; the volume of nursing delivered per unit/service; the nursing delivery unit/service accreditation; and the centralization of the environment of care delivery, which may be viewed as the extent to which decision-making power is distributed throughout the organization. Essential environmental variables also include the complexity of the clinical practice; the geographical accessibility of patients/clients; the method of care delivery

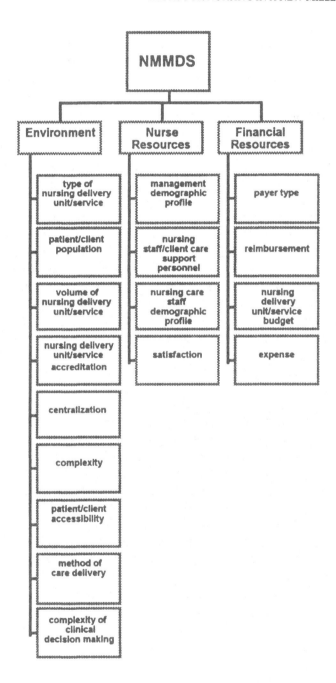

Figure 2.4. Nursing Management Minimum Data Set
SOURCE: Copyright D. Huber & C. Delaney.

employed, defined as the predominant method of organizing the delivery and accountability of care by the nursing unit/service; and the complexity of clinical decision making (Delaney & Huber, 1996).

Four essential variables are included in the *nurse resources* category. These describe the human resources aspects of delivering care to patients/clients. A description of the management demographic profile—which involves the demographics of the leadership of the nursing delivery unit/service and the demographics of the person, by whatever title, designated as the nurse manager with 24-hour administrative accountability over a nursing delivery unit/service; the nursing staff/client care support personnel; the nursing care staff demographic profile; and the satisfaction of all care and management nurse resources—composes a background of the people who provide the care (Delaney & Huber, 1996). The nurse manager can use the information derived from these elements to plan strategies that would enhance the human component of a service-intensive health care delivery system.

The final four elements of the NMMDS are grouped into the *financial resources* category. The payer type; reimbursement, defined as the distribution formula/payment for services within nursing delivery unit/service; nursing delivery unit/service budget; and expense variables provide the most basic data needs for describing the nursing unit/service level of resources (Delaney & Huber, 1996). Further aggregations are possible at broader organizational levels.

NMMDS APPLICATIONS TO PRACTICE

Nurse managers need data that are useable, accurate, timely, accessible, and quickly available. Administrative activities such as utilizing human resources, monitoring care provider competency, facilitating communication, and restructuring care delivery systems require efficient methods of managing and processing information (Romano, Mills, & Heller, 1996). Real-time information can be used in practice for performance enhancements and continuous quality and cost improvements. The NMMDS complements the nursing practice data available through implementation of the Nursing Minimum Data Set (NMDS) by providing for more precise decision making. Using NMMDS-generated data, nurses are empowered when challenged to justify resource expenditures and enhance outcomes. They can answer urgent practice questions. Further, by having access to sufficient and appropriate data, nurses can better formulate persuasive policy statements.

The NMMDS can be applied to nursing practice in four major ways. These applications include capturing consistent data for unit-/service-level decision making, providing a system for internal organizational benchmarking, creating the opportunity for external organizational benchmarking, and establishing a method of continuum of care evaluation (Huber, Schumacher, & Delaney, 1997). At last, nursing's added value to the health care improvements experienced by patients/clients can be made visible to nurses and their constituencies. Through the implementation of the NMMDS, nursing management variables can be linked to other relational databases and related "report card" systems.

REPORT CARD COMPARISONS

Quality monitoring and outcomes management have become imperatives with the movement to managed care. Payers have become increasingly interested in and demanding of data on quality indicators. These data may be a factor in signing managed care contracts. Along with internal quality improvement efforts, external quality reviews may or may not be a part of standardized performance reports, called "report cards."

A major standardized performance report is the Health Plan Employer Data and Information Set (HEDIS), which is widely used to measure the outcomes of managed health plans. There are more than 60 quality indicators in HEDIS version 2.5. The indicators sort into five broad categories: quality care, member access and satisfaction, membership and utilization, finance, and health plan management and activities. There are standard definitions and specifications for calculating the performance measures for comparability (Grimaldi, 1996). However, the 10 quality measures are all disease- or procedure- specific. Although a membership survey is used to capture information about member satisfaction with access and quality, other measures focus on physicians and their practices. Nursing data are obviously absent from HEDIS.

Within nursing a few data sets and performance measurement systems have been recommended. For example, DeGroot, Forsey, and Cleland (1992) displayed the Nursing Practice Personnel Data Set (NPPDS) for use in capturing human resources-related data in nursing. The American Nurses Association (ANA; 1995) published a nursing care report card that promulgated a nursing-sensitive quality and performance review set of elements. The NMMDS elements are mapped to the NPPDS and the ANA report card elements for comparison purposes in Table 2.1. The NMMDS focuses only on nursing management-specific essential data elements at the unit/service level. Thus, clinical practice or condition-specific elements do not map to the NMMDS variables and do not appear in the table. Table 2.1 clearly illustrates that the majority of key core contextual data needed for management decisions exist only in the NMMDS.

TABLE 2.1 NMMDS, ANA Report Card, and NPPDS Comparison

NMMDS	ANA	NPPDS
Type of nursing delivery unit/service		
Patient/client population		
Volume of nursing delivery unit/service	Total nursing care hours provided per patient (case mix, acuity adjusted)	
Nursing delivery care unit/ service accreditation		
Centralization		
Complexity		
Patient/client accessibility		
Complexity of clinical decision making		
Management demographic profile		(see demographics)
Nursing staff/client care support personnel		Position
Nursing care staff demographic profile	1. RN staff qualifications	1. Demographics
	2. Staff continuity	2. Professional education
	3. Nursing staff injury rate	3. Practice
	4. Ratio of RNs to total nursing staff	4. Organizational training
		5. Recruitment and retention
Satisfaction	1. Nurse satisfaction	
	2. Patient/family satisfaction with nursing care	
Payer type		
Reimbursement		
Nursing delivery unit/ service budget		
Expense	RN overtime	

SOURCE: Copyright D. Huber. Reprinted with permission.

The quality report card variables can be compared with the more traditional measures of quality. For example, the variables of falls, medication errors, skin breakdown, decubiti, patient complaints, nosocomial infections, mortality rate, and length of stay were selected for inclusion as the quality variables in Urden's (1996) decision support database. The traditional measures of "quality" represent broad measures of undesirable outcomes rather than quality. They are events that are not desired or that create risk. The NMMDS variables, however, seek to capture actual attributes of the environment, nurse resources, and financial resources that contribute to care delivery and coordination at the unit or service level as the lowest level of aggregation up from the individual patient/client. Implementation of the NMMDS will allow administrators to evaluate performance and quality in specific patient care or service units.

SUMMARY

The organization, management, and delivery of nursing and health care services to patients/clients is an information-intensive and information-dependent endeavor. Both performance and quality can be improved by developing management as well as clinical databases that are relational within broader information systems. Nurses and nurse managers can effect care management improvements by using the NMMDS for nursing management data capture. Being able to capture all elements of the NMMDS usually mandates changes in the design of both personnel and financial information systems. Nurses can influence the adaptation of technology to nursing's information needs. The result will be the coordination and integration of real-time interactive feedback from multiple departments and care providers. Such efforts are critical to patient/client care, demonstrating nursing effectiveness, and spotlighting the contributions of nursing practice to interdisciplinary health care delivery in the 21st century.

REFERENCES

American Nurses Association. (1995). *Nursing care report card for acute care.* Washington, DC: Author.

Anderson, R. A., Dobal, M. T., & Blessing, B. B. (1992). Theory-based approach to computer skill development in nursing administration. *Computers in Nursing, 10*(4), 152-157.

Axford, R. L., & Carter, B. E. L. (1996). Impact of clinical information systems on nursing practice: Nurses' perspectives. *Computers in Nursing, 14*(3), 156-163.

DeGroot, H. A., Forsey, L., & Cleland, V. S. (1992). The Nursing Practice Personnel Data Set. *Journal of Nursing Administration, 22*(3), 23-28.

Delaney, C., & Huber, D. (1996). *Nursing Management Minimum Data Set (NMMDS): A report of an invitational conference.* Chicago: American Organization of Nurse Executives.

Gates, B. (1995). *The road ahead.* New York: Viking Penguin.

Grimaldi, P. L. (1996, October). Monitoring managed care's quality. *Nursing Management,* Special suppl., *Managed care primer,* pp. 18-20.

Huber, D. G., Delaney, C., Crossley, J., Mehmert, P., & Ellerbe, S. (1992). A Nursing Management Minimum Data Set: Significance and development. *Journal of Nursing Administration, 22*(7/8), 35-40.

Huber, D., Schumacher, L., & Delaney, C. (1997). Nursing Management Minimum Data Set (NMMDS). *Journal of Nursing Administration, 27*(4), 42-48.

Iowa Intervention Project. (1996). *Nursing interventions classification (NIC)* (2nd ed.). St. Louis, MO: Mosby-Year Book.

Joint Commission on Accreditation of Healthcare Organizations (JCAHO). (1994). *1995 accreditation manual for hospitals: Vol. 1. Standards.* Oakbrook Terrace, IL: Author.

Jydstrup, R. A., & Gross, M. J. (1966). Cost of information handling in hospitals. *Health Services Research, 1*(3), 235-261.

Maas, M., Johnson, M., & Kraus, V. (1996). Nursing-sensitive patient outcomes classification. In K. Kelly (Ed.), *Outcomes of effective management practices* (Series on Nursing Administration, Vol. 8, pp. 20-35). Thousand Oaks, CA: Sage.

Maas, M., & Mulford, C. (1989). Structural adaptation of organizations. In M. Johnson (Ed.), *Changing organizational structures* (Series on Nursing Administration, Vol. 2, pp. 3-20). Menlo Park, CA: Addison-Wesley.

Martin, K., & Scheet, N. (1992). *The Omaha system: Applications for community health nursing.* Philadelphia: W. B. Saunders.

Morrison, R., & Keyes, R. (1989). Nursing management diagnosis. *Nursing Management, 20*(9), 23-24.

National Center for Nursing Research. (1992). Research priorities in nursing informatics. *Report of the Priority Expert Panel on Nursing Informatics.* Washington, DC: Department of Health and Human Services, National Institute of Health, National Center for Nursing Research.

North American Nursing Diagnosis Association (NANDA). (1994). *Nursing diagnosis: Definition and classification 1995-1996.* Philadelphia: Author.

Pew Health Professions Commission. (1995). *Critical challenges: Revitalizing the health professions for the twenty-first century.* San Francisco: UCSF Center for the Health Professions.

Richart, R. (1970). Evaluation of a medical data system. *Computers in Biomedical Research, 3*(5), 415-425.

Romano, C. A., Mills, M. E. C., & Heller, B. R. (1996). A conceptual basis for information management in nursing and health care. In M. E. C. Mills, C. A. Romano, & B. R. Heller (Eds.), *Information management in nursing and health care* (pp. 2-5). Springhouse, PA: Springhouse Corporation.

Ross, A. (1986). A Symposium on Contemporary Issues in Health Care: Integration of clinical and financial data systems. In B. J. Brown & A. Ross (Eds.), *Integration of clinical and financial information systems* (pp. xvii-xx). Rockville, MD: Aspen.

Saba, V. (1992). The classification of home health care nursing: Diagnoses and interventions. *Caring, 11,* 50-57.

Simpson, R. (1993). A Nursing Management Minimum Data Set. *Nursing Management, 24*(4), 24-25.

Tan, J. (1995). *Health management information systems.* Gaithersburg, MD: Aspen.

Urden, L. D. (1996). Development of a nurse executive decision support database: A model for outcomes evaluation. *Journal of Nursing Administration, 26*(10), 15-21.

Werley, H. H., & Lang, N. M. (Eds.). (1988). *Identification of the Nursing Minimum Data Set.* New York: Springer.

Wunderlich, G. S., Sloan, F. A., & Davis, C. K. (1996). *Nursing staff in hospitals and nursing homes: Is it adequate?* (Institute of Medicine). Washington, DC: National Academy Press.

Zielstorff, R. D., Hudgings, C. I., & Grobe, S. J. (1993). *Next generation nursing information systems: Essential characteristics for professional practice.* Washington, DC: American Nurses Association.

Zielstorff, R. D., McHugh, M. L., & Clinton, J. (1988). *Computer design criteria: For systems that support the nursing process.* Kansas City, MO: American Nurses Association.

CHAPTER 3

A Virtual Nursing Administration Collaboratory for Patient Outcomes Research

Linda Goodwin
Barbara Turner
Charlene Allred
Jack Yensen

Old paradigms of nursing administration are changing, as profit-driven motives and quality management principles bring data-driven and outcomes-focused decisions to health care. A new virtual paradigm is evolving, out of both opportunity and necessity, within a concept called a "collaboratory." A collaboratory is a virtual administrative meta-laboratory that connects multiple sites and tools with nurse administrators who interact electronically, using the Internet and the World Wide Web (WWW). Development of a Virtual Nursing Administration Collaboratory provides an opportunity for nurse administrators, from around the world, to communicate and collaborate in administrative problem solving, strategic planning, and outcomes research.

Progress toward a better understanding and linking between nursing actions and patient outcomes will be enhanced if collaborative sharing of data includes storing original raw data, and the interpretation(s) of that data, in a common format that can be readily compared with the results of other analyses and methodologies. Nurse administrators could contribute to the development of nursing's knowledge base by entering new data, generating appropriate methods of analysis and interpretation, comparing results, and facilitating the research-theory-practice link by disseminating validated scientific results into clinical practice patterns. This level of collaboration and data sharing will rely on tools much more sophisticated than traditional literature-search and database programs. Interactive development of collaboratory tools and shared data models will require the expertise of nurse administrators as well as advanced nursing informatics specialists and computer scientists. Common, extensible data models must be agreed upon, and standard tools for interacting with the data models must be created. Issues of data quality, privacy and confidentiality of patient data, and authentication of a participant's expertise are just a few of many issues that will require attention and resolution in collaboratory development. There are few models and mentors to guide this development, thus Virtual Nursing Administration Collaboratory development is a pioneering effort and a significant step forward to a fundamentally new way of doing both nursing administration and nursing science in the 21st century.

Old paradigms of scientific research are changing as funding becomes more competitive and less available, and as institutions demand more productivity of nursing administrators while decreasing both their numbers and their resources. A collaboratory is a virtual research meta-laboratory that connects multiple sites and tools with researchers who use the Internet and the World Wide Web (WWW) to interact electronically. Development of a Virtual Nursing Administration Research Collaboratory provides an opportunity for nurse administrators, from around the world, to communicate and collaborate with administrative colleagues, nurse scientists, and clinical practitioners in the process of complex problem solving.

Nursing is a compelling choice for collaboratory development. The task of health care reform, facing nations all around the globe, is enormous. Solutions will require integration of work in many fields, including nursing, that coordinates multiple complex studies and avoids unnecessary and expensive duplication. Because of the complexity in health care, chronicity, and humans' responses to their health and illness, progress in knowledge base development in nursing requires an ever-increasing synthesis of information from a variety of data sources and nurse experts. The links among data, patient problems, nursing interventions, and patient outcomes have yet to be articulated and evaluated. Collaboratory development establishes and supports an electronic community of nurse administrators who are researching and developing innovative solutions to problems related to illness care, health promotion, and outcomes research.

THE COLLABORATORY CONCEPT

The international computing infrastructure that supports collaboratory activity has developed rapidly and creates the opportunity for global cooperative and collaborative computing, using the World Wide Web. The World Wide Web (WWW or W3) began as a networked information project at CERN (the European Laboratory for Particle Physics) as a vision by Tim Berners-Lee (Berners-Lee, Cailliau, Groff, & Pollermann, 1992). Among the WWW's user-friendly techniques is a software technique called hypertext. Users who want more information about a particular subject in a hypertext document simply "click" on the subject topic to read further detail. Hypertext documents are often linked to other documents by completely different authors—much like footnoting—but the user gains immediate access to the referenced document! The WWW operates on a principle of "universal readership," which means that once information is made available in hypertext format, it should be accessible from any type of computer anywhere in the world for any user.

Software programs called "browsers" are used to access the WWW. Browsers read hypertext documents from a variety of sources. Hypermedia is similar to hypertext, but includes images, sound, movies, and animation in addition to text. Information providers set up hypertext and hypermedia servers from which browsers can search, view, and download documents. The documents that the browsers display are hypertext or hypermedia documents. The browsers let the user deal with the document links and pointers in a transparent way, such that the person may concentrate on the information provided and ignore the actual commands given to the computer to access the information. Netscape (http://home.netscape.com), Microsoft's Internet Explorer (http://www.microsoft.com), and others are extremely effective browser soft-ware programs that allow individuals to access the WWW and share distributed information. However, the user's interaction with the WWW using these browser tools is unidirectional, asynchronous, and limited to a client-server model in which a single user works with predefined data. Development efforts are in progress to augment the WWW for bidirectional and synchronous collaboration that exploits the WWW's ease of access and use, and incorporates a peer-to-peer model that provides real-time collaboration services. An exam-ple of this synchronous collaboration can be found in Microsoft's NetMeeting software (http://www.microsoft.com) that allows multiple people to dialogue using video, audio, and text-based technologies.

Client-server computing is based on modular programming concepts. With client-server architecture, the person requesting information becomes the "client," and the information that is being requested becomes the "server." The client uses a program module that sends a message to a server program module, requesting that the server perform a task or service. The client module is the front-end user interface of the application. Client workstations are considered user-friendly if they have a well-designed graphical user interface (GUI). The server module performs the back-end tasks that are common to similar applications, such as managing shared database resources, printers, communication links, or high-powered processors.

Global network connectivity and client-server architecture have changed our administrative landscape. Each networked computer resides within a local, regional, and global computer web rather than existing in isolation. As network and WWW connectivity become an integral part of computing systems, changes are required in our administrative processes to take advantage of global computing and research resources. Exploiting the resources fully, however, requires a paradigm shift away from old models in which an individual conducted research in a particular laboratory or setting, to new models of cooperation and collaboration among nurse administrators and nurse scientists who are distributed around the globe. New levels of cooperation and teamwork will be required to gain maximum benefit from a team of collaborators who share common goals in the study of patient outcomes. Reengineering outcomes research processes to take advantage of these benefits, from a global web of computers, creates various new opportunities and raises numerous issues.

Until the mid-1990s, use of the global computing network was manual and primitive, requiring sophistication and effort on the part of the end user to exploit the resources. Development of the WWW helped automate network use and make it user-friendly. Global cooperative computing represents the next step in exploiting WWW connectivity. Cooperative computing models, currently under development, support systems that continually adapt to end user needs and global information resources. This adaptability delivers considerable performance and convenience advantages for both developers and end users, and will be an essential component of reengineered research processes.

The National Research Council (USA) published a report titled *National Collaboratories, Applying Information Technology for Scientific Research* (Cerf et al., 1993) that described a collaboratory as a center without walls in which the nation's researchers can perform research without regard to geographical location—interacting with colleagues, accessing instrumentation, sharing data and computational resources, and accessing information from digital libraries. The report concluded that collaboratory test bed programs have the potential to address important scientific needs while simultaneously representing a key step toward developing national and global infrastructure. The collaboratory concept uses innovative new communication and information technologies to provide opportunities for improving ties among team members in a given research area, promoting collaborations among administrators and researchers in diverse areas, accelerating development and dissemination of new knowledge, and minimizing the time lag between discovery and application.

A successful collaboratory will require developments in computer communications and integration technologies for sharing data, programs, products, and ideas. Creation of a collaboratory culture based on methods of interacting with remote personnel and of accessing remote resources will have to be designed, developed, tested, and measured. Development of collaboratory research teams that acknowledge and value the benefits of electronic collaboration and the use of computer-based collaboration as a research tool will need to be investigated and implemented. Successful collaboratory development effort will also need a wide range of expertise to explore these areas. Success will also require tailoring the application of these technologies and cultures to the needs and wants of individual collaboratory team members.

It is the access to remote and unique research sites and instruments, as well as distributed interactions between people, that is the focus of the Virtual Nursing Administration Collaboratory for Patient Outcomes Research. The collaboratory test bed conducts studies related to the design, development, utilization, and evaluation of environments that support electronic team collaboration in patient outcomes research.

DEVELOPMENT OF THE VIRTUAL
NURSING ADMINISTRATION COLLABORATORY
FOR PATIENT OUTCOMES RESEARCH (VNARC)

The Virtual Nursing Administration Collaboratory for Patient Outcomes Research began, as a concept, in 1995. The goal of this collaboratory is to increase a nurse administrator's efficiency and productivity by leveraging nursing intellectual, financial, and physical resources related to patient outcomes research. To make the best use of resources, collaboratory development efforts should themselves be collaborative. Taking ownership of the process empowers collaboratory participants to develop projects and products that meet an individual administrator's needs and can be shared among colleagues.

The Virtual Nursing Administration Collaboratory for Patient Outcomes Research is based on concepts described by Wulf (1993) and consists of researchers who participate in research laboratories and patient outcomes research projects through WWW communication and collaboration. A nursing collaboratory will be most successful if it combines educational, theoretical, research, and nursing practice programs.

The initial goals identified for The Virtual Nursing Administration Collaboratory for Patient Outcomes Research follow:

1. To build an international electronic community of nurse administrators

2. To support patient outcomes research that defines and refines nursing knowledge and articulates links between nursing assessment, interventions, and patient outcomes

3. To support collaboratory participants both personally and professionally

4. To promote communication, cooperation, and collaboration that enhance research efforts and avoid redundancy and duplication of research efforts

5. To sponsor multisite replication that provides for highly cost-effective research extending into high statistical power and rapid implementation of findings

6. To identify and resolve issues that arise in collaboratory research and development efforts

7. To promote health and well-being for citizens of planet Earth

COLLABORATORY MODEL AND COMPONENTS

An underlying philosophical basis for collaboratory development is that the collaboratory should support nursing administration research that operates within a research-theory-practice paradigm in which all activities should contribute to enhancing and improving patient outcomes. Education is considered the vehicle that promotes and supports this practice-driven paradigm. Given that philosophical paradigm, the challenge for collaboratory development is to determine what infrastructure is needed to support it. The model (Figure 3.1) depicts the infrastructure components that include Distributed Systems Technology, WWW and Information Resources, User-Friendly Interfaces, Social Systems, and Pilot Projects. Each of these components will be discussed in further detail.

Distributed Systems Technology

The collaboratory functions in a distributed systems technology environment that includes the wide-area network of planet Earth. Virtual Nursing Administration Collaboratory success relies heavily on computer and communications technologies that will eventually allow connection by voice, video, text, virtual reality, and other innovations not yet designed. The evolving technologies will support remote research activities from a desktop workstation, where the team member can immediately access WWW information from all over the world. Information overload will be managed through personal "knowbots," or intelligent agents, that are programmed to search the WWW as both data producing filters and information producing filters for the collaborator's specified domain of inquiry. Thus, from a research laboratory or office anywhere in the world, a collaboratory team member can acquire raw

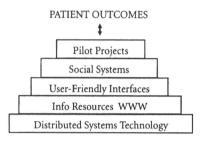

PATIENT OUTCOMES

Pilot Projects
Social Systems
User-Friendly Interfaces
Info Resources WWW
Distributed Systems Technology

Figure 3.1. Collaboratory Development Model

data, library resources, and other information from anywhere on the WWW, through his or her personalized intelligent agent software that does a lot of the tedious and time-consuming WWW searching without human intervention. The researcher's or administrator's time can be used to evaluate the quality of the found resources, rather than for searching for their existence.

Software tools required for development of a collaboratory include WWW browsers; data-sharing and data-mining tools; software that will permit instrumentation, computation, and observation from remote locations; and teleconferencing tools. Tools for requesting information and searching for collaborators improve upon the idea of e-mail, bulletin boards, and news groups. Desktop access to peer-reviewed literature is essential for a collaboratory, and digital libraries are currently working to resolve copyright issues for WWW dissemination of current literature. Enhancing literature access with hypertext capabilities for attaching comments to papers and exchanging informal notes with the authors could speed both the development and dissemination of new knowledge in nursing. While there are many issues that relate to client-server and distributed systems technology, it is important to understand that the technology exists now.

Information Resources

Nurses now have vastly expanded information resources. Traditional journals and textbooks are gradually being replaced with on-line, up-to-date digital libraries around the world. Personal knowbots can manage information by filtering the WWW's vast resources for searches that are specified (or programmed) to compile relevant resources at the local level for the nurse administrator's analysis and review. With proliferation of information servers on the WWW, the information available to nurses grows daily and in exponential volume. It is not humanly possible to manage the volume of information in any given domain, as it is now believed that knowledge doubles every few months. We have truly arrived at the "Information Age." The key to success, for both collaboratory and individual nurse administrators, will be to learn information processing strategies that filter the "best" information from that which is useless or of poorer quality. The plethora of information resources has become both the blessing and the curse of the new virtual paradigm, since filtering information (both with and without knowbots) is both tedious and time-consuming.

The World Wide Web (WWW)

Development of the WWW, discussed previously, includes concepts of high-performance computing and communications. The technology to support a global distributed systems environment and planetary information resources is foundational for nursing collaboratory development. Communication can take many forms (e-mail, listserv, postal mail, fax, voice telephone, and video-conferencing), but high-performance communication implies WWW transmission of all types of data/information using voice technology and video conferencing from small pocket-sized computers with wireless infrared transmission as these technologies are further developed. Traditional forms of communication have given way to e-mail and discussion lists, and collaboratory researchers are gradually moving toward group conferencing technologies, such as Microsoft's NetMeeting product, depicted in Figure 3.2.

Human (User-Friendly) Interfaces

User-friendly interfaces to access the WWW have already been developed and can be located and downloaded, sometimes without cost to the end user. These programs are called WWW "browsers"; an example is *Netscape*— (http://info@netscape.com). The sample collaboratory screens in this chapter were built and accessed using Netscape (version 3.0). User-friendly knowbot packages are at various stages of development and testing (as well as various stages of user-friendliness), and will become more readily available within the next few years. For an example of a "semi-intelligent" agent that can be tailored to the end user's preferences, see Pointcast's URL (http://www.pointcast.com) where users can decide what cities they want to monitor for weather, what money market funds they want to monitor for performance, and so forth.

The collaboratory infrastructure provides an ability to link high-performance computing hardware and software into concerted and easy-to-use research tools. From their desktop workstations, nurse administrators can access worldwide resources for library searching, data sharing, possible funding sources,

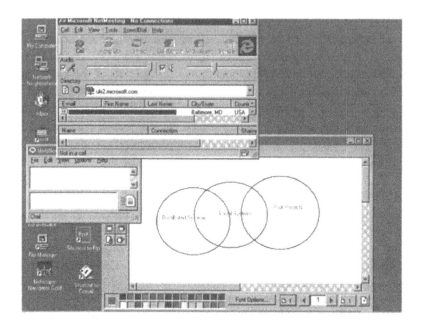

Figure 3.2. Microsoft NetMeeting (http://www.microsoft.com)

data analysis, experimental equipment, peer reviewers, and collaboration that is both synchronous and asynchronous with their colleagues. The sample screen in Figure 3.3 shows the first level of options that are available to collaboratory team members.

Each of the main selections takes the collaboratory team member to another screen with additional resources related to the chosen topic. The task of updating and maintaining the resource links is crucial to ongoing collaboration, collaboratory usage, and support for nurse administrators as they work toward solutions to the complex problems in nursing and patient outcomes research.

Nurse administrators utilize a wide variety of seemingly disparate experimental techniques to conduct outcomes studies and understand the links among data, nursing interventions, and patient outcomes. While common data sets are important in nursing, little has been done to share and exploit nursing databases. Comparison of raw data obtained from one patient system by two or more different analysis techniques is nontrivial. Both the raw data and the assumptions and algorithms used in their analysis affect the interpretation. Progress toward a better understanding and linking between nursing interven-

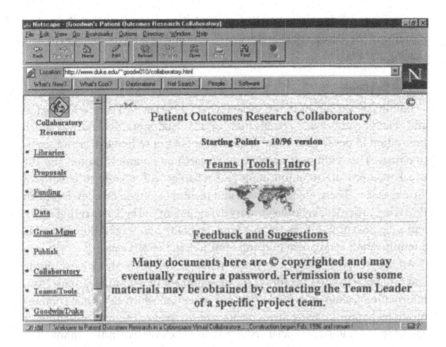

Figure 3.3. Collaboratory WWW Access/Entry Screen (http://www.duke.edu/goodw010)

tions and patient outcomes will be enhanced if collaborative sharing of data includes storing original raw data and the interpretation(s) of that data in a common format that can be readily compared with the results of other analyses and methodologies. Nurse administrators could contribute to the development of a nursing knowledge base by entering new data, generating appropriate methods of analysis and interpretation, comparing experimental results, and facilitating the research-theory-practice link by disseminating validated scientific results into clinical practice patterns.

This level of collaboration and data sharing will rely on tools much more sophisticated than traditional literature-search and database programs. Nurse administrators and other collaboratory team members will want to communicate with each other and discuss their data using teleconferencing, images, sound, whiteboards, and shared programs. Interactive development of collaboratory tools and shared data models will require the expertise of advanced nursing informatics specialists and computer scientists. Common, extensible data models must be agreed upon, and standard tools for interacting with the data models must be created. New opportunities for "telementoring" will find

experienced collaboratory participants assisting novices with their understanding of the virtual collaboratory paradigm and new methodologies of data
sharing and analysis.

Social Systems

Building a collaboratory is a social (Schatz, 1992) as well as a technological
and scientific endeavor. The creation of a collaboratory demands as much
innovation in developing social systems as it does in technological and scientific ones. The traditional methods of research and administration, and the
usual methods of communicating and relating, will operate differently in
virtual spaces. There are few models and mentors to guide this development;
thus it is anticipated that collaboratory development will be a pioneering effort,
and a significant step forward to a fundamentally new way of doing nursing
administration and patient outcomes research in the 21st century.

Anthropologists believe it was early humans' need to collaborate in hunting
and foraging activities that drove the development of communications. Now,
information technologies establish social systems in which electronic communications permit humans to cooperate and thrive, even though proximity is
absent in the traditional social systems sense. The ever-expanding innovation
and power of information technologies brings us all to the threshold of this
strange new collaboratory setting. In this manufactured, "virtual" place, where
space and time are maintained through loops of electronic information flow,
nurse administrators and collaboratory team members will convene, converse,
and cooperate on some of the most challenging health care problems of the
21st century. The collaboratory concept has already been proven technically
feasible in non-nursing domains.[1] The question is whether or not it is socially
sustainable in nursing administration and patient outcomes research projects.
Is it possible electronically to create a distributed team of nurse administrators
and collaborators that permits and even enhances the successful cooperation
of dispersed individuals toward common goals? The collaboratory's purpose is
to help structure inquiry, and this purpose can best be achieved through
successful development of collaboratory social systems.

Remote electronic communication with colleagues is a universal need for
collaboratory progression. Collaboratory communications tools are developing beyond voice and electronic mail to allow nurse administrators jointly to
visualize data and to share interaction with the data. This implies interactive
whiteboards, joint program control, and annotation overlay capabilities. These
are similar to the ways data are manipulated and discussed by researchers in
the same room. Since facial expressions and body language are major components of communicating, high-quality video connections among collaborators

should promote both the formal and informal relationships that are needed for successful collaboratory research. Collaboratory tools must also provide for spontaneous meetings and will, ideally, transmit the emotional content of communications. The electronic equivalent of hallway meetings is needed to allow collaboratory team members to exchange ideas safely that are not yet well formulated; these informal exchanges are safer among friends. The collaboratory creates the opportunity to develop virtual friendships. Will virtual friendships foster the kind of support that enhances nursing administrators in their work? Will virtual teams level the playing field so that interdisciplinary collaboration becomes authentic with our non-nursing colleagues? The amount of effort required to make interactions informal, useful, and productive is expected to vary with the individuals involved and their personal and professional values. Use of collaboratory tools, such as Microsoft's NetMeeting (see Figure 3.2), which can be downloaded from http://www.microsoft.com, provides an opportunity for group interaction and collaboration, regardless of geographic location.

As in traditional systems, the social aspects of collaboratory development and research will make or break the success of specific projects. The ability to develop formal working teams and informal friendships will depend on an ability to develop a common sense of purpose. Basic values of honesty, integrity, openness, tolerance, respect, trust, and more, will provide an environment that enhances rapid team development and research productivity. Nurses as a group, however, have not been consistently socialized to adopt and cultivate these values in their professional practice, and oppressed group behaviors (Roberts, 1996) create numerous problems for team efforts in general, and collaboratory team development in particular. Resolving issues of oppressed group behaviors, as well as of dispersed team members and project resources, creates a need and an opportunity for managing collaboratory teams differently than traditional project management.

Managing collaboratory development will use continuous quality improvement and teamwork strategies that include the participants in all aspects of process, system, and outcome analysis. Management strategies are needed that combine team members' ideas with knowledge of existing and possible technologies, and a knowledge of working collaboratory projects in other domains. The process is iterative and requires time and effort on the part of participating nurse administrators, nursing informatics specialists, and collaboratory team leaders. Other more general concerns will be addressed as well: How might collaboration be made attractive to nurse administrators? How should funding for collaborative work be administered? How will interdisciplinary projects be managed? How will credit for collaborative work accrue to individual participants? Development of a Virtual Nursing Administration Collaboratory for Patient Outcomes Research provides an opportunity to explore these issues through nontraditional agreements among collaborators.

Management strategies for collaboratory teams include a keen awareness of the value of social systems aspects in successful research projects. Technology and research do not operate in a vacuum, and often succeed or fail based upon the social systems into which they are introduced. Nursing collaboratory teams understand this phenomenon and work closely with current and potential nurse administrators to develop and sustain social systems that support and promote the goals and objectives of individual nurse administrators as well as the collaboratory at large. Management strategies to develop patient outcomes research teams include front-loading teams with knowledgeable, talkative, and diverse personalities who can stimulate scholarly discussion of ideas and sustain the teams through periods of disagreement and conflict. The nursing collaboratory teams are addressing social systems by front-loading teams with already active WWW users who share the basic values described above and who are "talkative," diverse, and tolerant while generating provocative discussions. There is a developing sense of community and "belonging" that will be important to sustain as further social systems develop within the collaboratory.

COLLABORATORY DEVELOPMENT ISSUES

Various issues arise when new modes of communicating and collaborating are made available through the Virtual Nursing Administration Collaboratory for Patient Outcomes Research. Some of the issues and challenges in the development of the collaboratory are clear; others will only surface once the effort has progressed further. Issues include the reliability of technology, the authentication of data and expertise, autonomy, trust, and myriad related issues that will be discussed further. Awareness of the issues is an important place to begin, and nurse administrators will acknowledge that many of these issues also exist outside the collaboratory. Answers and solutions are works-in-progress.

Hardware and software reliability issues are crucial to collaboratory development because collaboratory teams cannot communicate and collaborate when WWW links and transmissions fail. While of concern, these issues are in the computer science domain more than the nursing domain. Nursing informatics specialists, who have expertise in computer science and information science as well as nursing, can bridge the hardware and software issues of technology that impact nursing administration collaboratory research and development. Nursing informatics specialists, as well as computer scientists, will also address issues of interoperability. While the WWW has created an environment that is cross-platform and user-friendly, much of the data and software that will be available for nursing administrators will be platform specific. Interoperability issues that address the need to migrate and share data, programs, and so on, from PC to Macintosh to UNIX workstations, and others, will be addressed as a part of collaboratory development.

Another important issue is one of verification or authentication. If virtual collaboration is to proliferate, it will be necessary to ensure that electronically shared data provided is accurate, reliable, and valid. Security and confidentiality issues related to patient data exist, as in all research modes, but security and confidentiality of methodologies and tools that secure competitive funding will also arise. Issues of "ownership" (both of data and of ideas) must be dealt with. The people issues—(un)willingness to share and collaborate—involve monumental tasks in nursing that will be difficult to resolve in some situations. Also, it will be important to verify or authenticate the expertise and credentials of a potential collaborator.

Autonomy has been an issue for nurses since the proliferation of debate about whether or not nursing is a true profession (Styles, 1982). Autonomy, from a collaboratory standpoint, can be either a focal issue or a nonissue. The collaboratory depends on cooperation and external funding sources for survival; it is not a self-sustaining autonomous organization. However, individual nurse administrators who work within the collaboratory infrastructure consider themselves (and their colleagues) to be autonomous agents who come together voluntarily to achieve shared goals. The management strategies for the Virtual Nursing Administration Collaboratory for Patient Outcomes Research treat collaboratory participants as autonomous agents who are responsible and accountable for their own work. The collaboratory is simply the place where autonomous agents may choose to collaborate and coordinate their efforts to enhance their productivity. There is no hierarchical organizational chart and no sense of superior/subordinate among the collaboratory teams.

Virtual cooperative work will make progress on a basis of trust and, conversely, where trust does not develop, it is unlikely that virtual projects will succeed. Trust, in the collaboratory sense, includes learning to trust the technology. Trust of technology will develop as nurse administrators experience reliable performance, rapid fixes for technical problems, and user-friendly (intuitive) applications that enhance their work. The more difficult issues of trust are those between the people involved in collaboratory research and development. Trust between people is achieved through values and behaviors of honesty, integrity, and openness. Yet how is trust to be established among collaborators who may never meet face-to-face and who have little familiarity with a potential collaborator's personal values and professional behaviors? Clearly, developing trust among collaboratory participants will prove one of the most challenging tasks for collaboratory development. First steps in the process of getting to know collaboratory colleagues involves reviewing on-line biographical sketches (with pictures and personal histories) and development of electronic discussion groups for informal dialogue and "thinking aloud" with other nurse administrators who share common research interests. But this is only the beginning. Virtual Nursing Administration Collaboratory for Patient Outcomes Research projects will explore whether videoconferencing or synchronous multiple user discussions and other technologies help foster trust and cooperation among collaboratory participants.

It is not yet known if the Virtual Nursing Administration Collaboratory for Patient Outcomes Research can create a sense of location where individual nurse administrators feel they "belong." In the traditional health care setting, the nurse administrator is identified with his or her institution. This sense of belonging should remain intact for collaboratory participants, but will the collaboratory also create a new identity in which one "belongs" to this virtual sense of place? Having a sense of place can mean several things: It can mean being unique from other places, or it can mean an image that is visually recalled. Physical settings can foster a multitude of emotional and intellectual responses among a group of collaborators. Will this also be true of virtual settings? If a collaboratory can harness some of the design strategies that have been so successful in physical group settings, it may also create a sense of place and purpose among its dispersed members that will engender an enduring sense of affiliation and cooperation toward shared goals. Creation of a sense of place may be important for Virtual Nursing Administration Collaboratory for Patient Outcomes Research development because it is expected that this will influence attitudes, interactions, and relationships among collaboratory participants.

Educating users and potential users creates issues and challenges for collaboratory development. Educational programs need to inform nurses about ever-changing collaboratory resources and opportunities. Keeping both the resources and educational programs about those resources current will prove to be a labor-intensive task. Who will perform this ongoing task, and who will pay for it? Nurse administrators will need to understand (and endorse) the benefits of collaborative work to their organizations. They will need to learn new methods for supporting and managing employees who are engaged in collaborative research, development, and maintenance. Developing and maintaining a collaboratory effort will prove difficult without a high level of commitment and cooperation from nurse administrators.

Pilot Projects

Searchable hypermedia databases are being developed to provide text, images, sound, movies, and animation that describe both the potential collaborators and their work. An "idea gallery" is under construction to enable nurse administrators to engage in sharing ideas with each other, with non-nursing health care administration colleagues, with nurse educators and researchers, and with nurses in clinical practice. This idea gallery will be a place to clarify problems and questions, compare theoretical and practical aspects of diverse projects, discuss data analysis results, disseminate research findings, and more. Ultimately, our body of knowledge in nursing is practice-driven by, and our knowledge development research activities need close links to, patients and the nurses who provide their care.

Global cooperative computing and wide-area interoperable databases with large volumes of clinical data will be used for pilot projects to collect problems, interest, and coordinate distributed optimization and search. Individual nurse scientists will use technology, both individually and collectively, to work on health care problems and to communicate the results to the profession through the Virtual Nursing Administration Research Collaboratory. Dissemination of research findings is more rapid than traditional methods, and the findings become part of the worldwide knowledge base.

Pilot work involves iterative development, prototyping, and research elements that help define and refine the work of collaboratory participants. Shared problem solving, shared data, shared analyses and interpretations, and shared manuscript development are ongoing activities for Virtual Nursing Administration Collaboratory for Patient Outcomes Research collaborators. On-line WWW consultation saves travel time and money, and permits expert consultation even on limited budgets. Pilot projects are selected for their potential contribution within a nursing research-theory-practice paradigm. The initial list of pilot projects begun in 1996 includes the following:

1. Perinatal outcomes research among Duke University, the University of Kansas, the University of Missouri, and the University of Virginia. This is a funded project (PI—Linda Goodwin, National Library of Medicine—1RO1LM/NRO6468-01) that seeks to predict preterm birth outcomes from large clinical databases.

2. Skin care and ARDS outcomes research between nurses and nurse administrators at Duke University (USA) and in Vienna (Austria). This is a Hewlett-Packard Corporation-funded project that seeks to predict patients at risk for ARDS and to examine the effectiveness of positioning on patient outcomes.

3. Advanced nursing practice influence on a variety of patient outcome measures in a psychiatric-mental health specialty throughout Duke University's integrated delivery system. This is an internally funded project at Duke University that seeks

to explicate and define advanced nursing practice for purposes of developing documentation systems across numerous divisions and departments.

OPPORTUNITIES

The Virtual Nursing Administration Collaboratory for Patient Outcomes Research provides opportunities for nurse administrators to be more productive through cooperation and collaboration. Research is strengthened through multisite replication. Expanded social systems networking creates a community of nurse administrators who exchange ideas and provide professional and personal support for individual participants. Improved communication and collaboration minimize duplication and redundancy, such that knowledge development in an individual participant's work builds on an already publicized domain (where one exists), or communicates to the nursing collaboratory teams that a new domain of knowledge building is now in progress. Knowledge domains will be mapped, and links identified and described, to help articulate a coherent body of nursing knowledge. Incremental and supplemental knowledge building that is scrutinized by international nursing collaboratory participants (in the spirit of cooperation and collaboration) will help define and advance the important links between nursing and patient outcomes.

SUMMARY AND CONCLUSIONS

Collaboratories have the potential to benefit nursing greatly by expanding the resources available to individual nurse administrators, and offer a new paradigm of developing, conducting, and disseminating solutions. The collaboratory concept is a qualitatively different way of using communication and information technologies to solve complex problems in health care. Collaboratories will create a new paradigm "meta-laboratory" with capabilities—in both expertise and technology—that far exceed those available in any one institution. Whether or not the Virtual Nursing Administration Collaboratory for Patient Outcomes Research will succeed depends on the development of trust within social systems, resolution of numerous issues, and sustaining energy and momentum for innovative collaboratory nurse administrators.

NOTE

1. Readers are encouraged to use their favorite WWW search engines in finding "collaboratory" examples in space research, environmental research, K-12 education, medical education and research, and many other areas.

REFERENCES

Berners-Lee, T., Cailliau, R., Groff, J.-F., & Pollermann, J. (1992). World-Wide Web: The information universe. *Electronic Networking, 2*(1), 52-58.

Cerf, V. G., et al. (1993). *National collaboratories, applying information technology for scientific research.* Washington, DC: National Academy Press.

Roberts, S. J. (1996). Breaking the cycle of oppression. *Journal of the American Academy of Nurse Practitioners, 8*(5), 209-214.

Schatz, B. R. (1992). Building an electronic community system. *Journal of Management Information Systems, 8*(3), 87-107.

Styles, M. (1982). *On nursing: Toward a new endowment.* St. Louis, MO: C. V. Mosby.

Wulf, W. A. (1993). The collaboratory opportunity. *Science, 261*(5123), 854-855.

PART II

Strategies for an
Information Revolution

This section focuses on basic skills and strategies for nurse administrators who are entering the information age. The chapters provide basic content and "how to" information on a variety of technology advancements affecting nursing practice and health care delivery.

In the first chapter of this section, Shellenbarger and Zuraikat highlight a variety of electronic resources that can be used to support nursing practice, education, administration, and research. In a user-friendly approach, the authors identify the equipment and software that are required and the electronic resources available, and conclude with a discussion of educational activities required to use these technologies. Specifically, the authors discuss electronic mail, discussion and news groups, library information services, on-line journals, and marketing and recruitment resources.

Scherb, in Chapter 5, describes a strategy for enhancing employee performance evaluations. This strategy focuses on using information that is already gathered within a computerized information system to enhance objectivity, minimize bias, and increase the reliability and validity of data used in the evaluation process. For example, the author highlights the derivation of an individual nurse profile from implementation of the Nursing Minimum Data Set. The profile may highlight the types of patients the nurse cares for over a period of time, including nursing diagnoses, interventions, and outcomes. She further proposes enhancing performance evaluation by linking this nurse care profile to data concerning professional development activities.

In Chapter 6, Kellum and Tatum provide a basic overview of administrative, clinical, and educational applications in health care information technology. The authors clearly emphasize the necessity for developing and implementing interactive systems in all of these areas and discuss the foundations of this change. This chapter is recommended for managers and administrators who are in the process of implementing a nursing information system in their setting.

In Chapter 7, Ireson and Velotta describe a strategy to increase nurses' accessibility to current, completed research for use in clinical practice. This chapter presents an insightful use of Rogers's model of infusion and adoption of technology of an innovation. The content focuses on research utilization and use of the computer to increase the nurses' access to research-based knowledge.

An additional strategy for increasing research utilization in practice is described in the final chapter in this section. Layman, Funk, and Cobb highlight how the Center for Research on Chronic Illness shared research through the World Wide Web. Specifically, the authors describe how Web pages were developed, the costs involved, the strategies for evaluating and maintaining the pages, and the methods for publicizing this resource. This application may stimulate others to use this technology to ensure that research utilization is indeed responsive to the quickly changing health care environment and nursing practice.

CHAPTER 4

Electronic Communication and Computer Linkages for Nurse Managers

Teresa Shellenbarger
Nashat Zuraikat

As computer technology continues to expand rapidly, nurses need to increase their awareness and understanding of available electronic communication and computer capabilities. This chapter describes how nurses can use computers and Internet access as a valuable resource tool.

A brief description of the Internet is provided as well as an introduction to gaining Internet access, with instructions for using electronic mail as a method of communication. Information on discussion and news groups is also provided.

Because the Internet provides a wealth of on-line clinical information important for nurses and managers in the practice setting, gaining access to library resources, conducting searches, and subscribing to on-line journal information is described. The chapter proceeds with a description of how the Internet can be used to obtain information about funding and grant resources, as well as how nurses can use the Internet for marketing and recruitment issues. The chapter ends with information about continuing education opportunities using the computer and the Internet.

Advances in technology have created an explosion of information and communication networks. Students, from elementary to graduate school, are using computers in the classroom. The Internet is becoming an important business tool. Traditionally, nurse managers have used computers for staffing, scheduling, patient classification, nursing workload calculations, budgeting activities, office automation, and other record-keeping activities (Ball, Hannah, Newbold, & Douglas, 1995; Haynor & Wells, 1992; Saba, Johnson, & Simpson, 1994). However, new opportunities for various computer usage now exist through the Internet and the World Wide Web. Nurse leaders and other health care providers must begin to use computers to keep up with the current knowledge and technological explosion and consider the new technology as an essential resource for their roles.

Computer experts suggest that "those who don't have access to computers and networks will be highly correlated with the general have nots" (Simpson, 1995, p. 18). This chapter will assist nurses to develop a better understanding of the Internet, the World Wide Web, electronic communication, and the use of computer linkages for nursing purposes.

THE INTERNET

The Internet is one area of recent computer growth. "The number of Internet users has increased a thousandfold (now estimated at 15-20 million) in the past seven years" (Tietze & Huber, 1995, p. 36). Estimates suggest that more than 10,000 people subscribe to Internet services every day, although it is difficult to get an accurate count because growth is occurring so rapidly (Griffith, 1996).

The Internet is frequently described as a "network of networks," because thousands of computers connect through a network (DuBois & Rizzolo, 1994; Kehoe, 1994; Nicoll, 1994b; Tietze & Huber, 1995). Users can communicate with or use the services located on any of these networked computers. Although the Internet has experienced rapid growth recently, it was initiated more than 25 years ago as a U.S. Department of Defense experiment (Edwards, 1995; Wink, 1995). It has expanded to more than "34,000 networks, five million computers, and 20 million users" (Nicoll, 1994b, p. 9).

GETTING STARTED

Nurses need to understand the hardware and software components to begin using electronic communication. Hardware is the actual computer equipment: the monitor, the keyboard, and any other peripheral equipment. Software is what allows the hardware to work by telling the computer hardware what to do (Saba, 1994; Saba, Johnson, & Simpson, 1994). Software, also known as the computer program, operates the computer (Joos, Whitman, Smith, & Nelson, 1992). Communication software allows computers to interact with each other.

The Internet requires computers to communicate so that exchange of information occurs via the networks. One way this is accomplished is by utilizing a modem and a telephone line. The modem is a hardware device that allows the transmission of data via the phone lines by converting digital signals to an analog form (Joos et al., 1992). Modems can be external, connected to a serial port on the computer, or internal, connected inside the computer hardware in an expansion slot. When purchasing a modem, the fastest modem affordable should be selected. Wink (1995) suggests a 14,400-baud minimum modem for Internet use.

Hardware, software, and a modem still are not sufficient to allow Internet access; an Internet access provider is also needed. The Internet access provider allows for the transfer of information via a standard protocol, usually known as Transmission Control Protocol/Internet Protocol (TCP/IP) (Nicoll, 1994b).

There are two methods of gaining Internet access, direct and indirect. The first involves a direct computer connection with a network device known as an Ethernet card, thereby eliminating the modem. More commonly, Internet users access a computer that creates an indirect connection with TCP/IP (Nicoll, 1994b; Tomaiuolo, 1995).

There are a variety of ways to gain indirect Internet access. One method is to use a gateway established by a company, university, or hospital (Edwards, 1995). The gateway usually allows the user to access the Internet free of charge. The user has a limited connection to the Internet through a modem and a remote terminal computer. The user's computer connects to a TCP/IP-connected computer.

Some cities around the United States have a community-based system that allows Internet access, such as the Denver Free-Net or the Cleveland Free-Net. Citizens in these communities can access the Internet, although the service availability may be limited.

A third method for gaining indirect Internet access involves commercial providers that offer various types and ranges of services at different prices, depending upon options selected (Marine, Kirkpatrick, Neou, & Ward, 1994). Three major on-line service providers are America Online, Prodigy, and Compuserve (Ayre, 1995). Many Internet providers have flat fee plans costing about $25 per month. Others may charge an hourly fee based on the amount of on-line time used (Ayre, 1995); the fee may be compounded with long distance charges if the provider number is not a local call. The commercial providers may provide a SLIP (Serial Line Internet Protocol) or a PPP (Point-to-Point

Protocol) connection, thus providing a gateway to the Internet (Edwards, 1995).

ACCESSING INTERNET INFORMATION

There are a variety of programs that provide access to information on the Internet, including Gopher, Telnet, and the World Wide Web. Gopher is a program that allows Internet users to select items for display from an on-screen menu. This menu eliminates the need to recall specific address information for electronic resources (DuBois & Rizzolo, 1994).

Telnet, another computer program, provides a route for connecting to remote computers. After logging in, access can be gained to the resources provided by the host computer. The *American Journal of Nursing* is a host that allows others to access its computer system, by using Telnet, with their on-line address <ajn.org>.

The World Wide Web (WWW or Web) is also an information retrieval system available via networked computers. It allows the user to select links to other sites. The Web user can move from site to site by selecting specially marked hypertext. The hypertext link format also allows the display of text in graphic and audio form. This linking capability distinguishes the Web from the traditional linear format of the gopher or Telnet. Web browser software packages are needed for World Wide Web access. Software packages such as Mosaic (freeware) or Netscape (Netscape Communications Corp.) allow interpretation and display of the graphic hypertext Web documents.

The first page of a WWW document is known as the home page (see Figure 4.1). Home pages are becoming the 1990's equivalent of business cards, sales brochures, and/or personal résumés. Addresses for Web home pages are found by using the Uniform Resource Locator (URL), which contains two parts. The first part is the access method for the file, such as http (hypertext transmission protocol). The second part consists of the address of the desired information to be retrieved, such as www.ajn.org.

Regardless of the access method selected, users of the Internet and the World Wide Web can obtain large amounts of text, video, or audio material in seconds. These Internet files can be transferred by file transfer protocol (FTP) and downloaded to the user's computer. Since the Internet is growing so large, novice users may have difficulty finding appropriate resources on the Internet. Many browsers offer a search option that allows for terms to be matched to Internet resources. There are also search engines such as Yahoo <http://www.yahoo.com> and AltaVista <http://www.altavista.digital.com/> that record Internet information for easy search and retrieval.

IUP Nursing Home Page

Welcome to the home page of Indiana University of Pennsylvania (IUP), Department of Nursing and Allied Health. The IUP nursing program is part of the IUP College of Health and Human Services. Other majors in the college include: Food and Nutrition, Health and Physical Education, Hotel, Restaurant, and Institutional Management, Human Development and Environmental Studies, and Safety Sciences.

The IUP nursing program is approved by the state board of nursing and is fully accredited by the National League of Nursing.

This page includes

- The <u>history</u> of the department.
- <u>The Nursing Faculty at IUP</u>. This is a listing of the various graduate and undergraduate nursing faculty. It also contains detailed information about select members of the nursing faculty.
- <u>BS</u>
- <u>MS</u>
- <u>Other Nursing Sites On the Web</u> Finding other sites on the Internet dealing with the nursing profession.
- <u>Organizations and Activities</u> within the Department of Nursing at IUP.

 This site is currently under construction. Thank you all for your patience.

Figure 4.1. Home Page Example

ELECTRONIC MAIL

Once on-line access has been gained, users will want to learn how to use electronic mail, the most widely used Internet application (Kehoe, 1994; Levine & Young, 1994). Electronic mail (e-mail) is a method of communicating via the computer by which the sender transmits a message electronically to the recipient's "mailbox." The recipient can read the mail at any convenient time, save it, delete it, reply to it, forward it to someone else, or discard it, just as can be done with traditional mail.

There is a standard structure for mail messages and mail addresses, which generally includes a header and a body. The header usually contains information such as return address and time of mailing. The body contains the text of the mail message. All electronic mail users have an address that consists of the user (the account or user name) followed by a system or location where the mail account is found, such as a university, company, government site, or private organization. Mail addresses may also have a country code for users such as "ca" for Canada or "au" for Australia. This information is combined in a standard format that all e-mail users will recognize. For example, the author can be reached at the following electronic mail address: <tshell@grove. iup.edu>—meaning that user "tshell" has an account on the "grove system" at "IUP" (Indiana University of Pennsylvania), an educational ("edu") institution. Another e-mail address could be <shell@prodigy.com>, meaning that the user has an account on Prodigy, a commercial server.

Anderson (1992) suggests that electronic mail is advantageous for organizations because it increases the productivity of the workers. Electronic mail allows nurses to communicate more rapidly and efficiently with colleagues, co-workers, and supervisors regarding policy information, changes in procedures, or other administrative information.

Electronic mail communication is important because it is rapid, with the mail message appearing almost instantly in the recipient's mailbox. It is also convenient because timing is not an issue; a message can be sent at 8:00 in the morning or 11:00 at night. Electronic mail is always available. Mail can be sent to any networked computer user within a corporation or anywhere around the world. Users do not lose time because of the need for repeated contact, delays, or interruptions that might occur when trying to communicate via traditional phone lines.

Electronic mail can be useful for nurse managers by facilitating collaboration with other professionals in other institutions. Nurses may also save time by conducting electronic meetings by using e-mail. Electronic mail also allows nurses to function more effectively by creating an electronic distribution list that allows the nurse to send mail to all list members. When the nurse sends a message to the list, it is automatically distributed to all members on that list.

Certain problems may occur when using electronic mail and distribution lists for communication. For example, if others are not on-line or do not check their mail routinely, they may miss important messages. It is imperative that employees have access to computers, be encouraged to use this method of communication, and receive adequate training and opportunity for practice.

DISCUSSION GROUPS AND NEWS GROUPS

Discussion groups provide another forum for communication via the Internet. A discussion group is a group of people who communicate electronically

TABLE 4.1 Discussion Group Etiquette Guidelines

Save instructions for later reference

Send subscription requests to the listserv address

Determine if a reply should be sent to an individual reader or to the entire group

Send replies to the group to the mailserv address

Consider joining one discussion group at a time to evaluate the volume and content of the messages for the group

After initially subscribing, consider lurking (listening) to the group to learn about the tone and topic of conversations before posting messages or replies

Type messages in all caps for emphasis only; this usually implies shouting

Use correct spelling, grammar, and punctuation in all messages

about a specific topic via a group forum. Members of the discussion group can ask questions, raise issues, or share information with other members by posting an electronic mail message to a list address. The "listserv" program sends the message to all subscribers in the group. Usually, a discussion group will have a manager who adds subscribers to the list (Levine & Young, 1994).

If consideration is being given to subscribing to a discussion group, general rules of etiquette should be followed. Refer to Table 4.1 for discussion group etiquette guidelines. Table 4.2 provides a list of discussion groups and addresses that might be helpful for nurse managers and those in clinical practice (Edwards, 1995; Gonzalez & Seaton, 1995). Subscription requests may be sent via electronic mail to the list address found in Table 4.2, with a message requesting subscription to the group and the user's name.

Discussion groups can be advantageous for nurse managers and practicing nurses. The discussion group allows for networking with colleagues around the globe. For example, in January 1996 a nursing education discussion group had more than 700 subscribers in 22 countries (Lacefield, 1996). Discussion groups can help answer questions or provide input/resources not available within the user's institution. At the present time there is no formal established discussion group for nurse managers, but that may change as more people begin to use this electronic communication method.

Nurse managers can have real-time discussions with other Internet users by accessing chat rooms on the World Wide Web. Guest speakers or others with similar interests can simultaneously interact and discuss issues of interest through these WWW chat rooms.

Nurse managers may also gain access to news information and messages about management topics via a news group. Messages about particular topics

TABLE 4.2 Nursing and Health Care Discussion Groups

Directions for subscribing to a discussion group: Send an electronic message to the address for
the discussion group listed below. In the message, type <discussiongroupname usersfirstname
userslastname>

Cancer Related issues (CANCER-L)
    listserv@wvnvm.wvnet.edu

CULTURE-AND-NURSING
    majordomo@itssrvll.ucsf

Geriatric health care discussion group
    gerinet@ubvm.cc.buffalo.edu

Health Research (HEALTH-L)
    listserv@irlean.ucd.ie

Health Resources (HMATRIX-L)
    listserv@ukanaix.cc.ukans.edu

IV therapy nursing (Ivtherapy-L)
    majordomo@netcome.com

International Research Project on Diabetes (DIABETES)
    listserv@irlean.ucd.ie

Medical Technology (MED-TECH)
    listserv@vm1.ferris.edu

Midwife discussion group (MIDWIFE)
    midwife@csv.warwick.ac.uk

Nursenet (nursing issues) discussion group
    nursenet@vm.utcc.utoronto.ca

Nursing research discussion group
    nurseres@kentvm.bitnet

Psychiatric-Nursing
    mailbase@mailbase.ac.uk

PUBLIC-HEALTH
    mailbase@mailbase.ac.uk

Research in fetal and perinatal care (FET-NET)
    listserv@hearn.bitnet

RURALNET-L
    listserv@musom01.mu.wvnet.edu

Telecommunications in healthcare (CPRI-L)
    listserv@ukanaix.cc.ukans.edu

or themes are posted to a news group just as a message might be placed on a
bulletin board. The reader can then visit the bulletin board and read the notes
posted to the group rather than having the mail messages sent directly to a
mailing list. Usenet is an Internet system of news groups that contains general
areas of interest as well as highly specialized topics, such as information about
ulcerative colitis. News groups are constantly being created, with more than

10,000 news groups in existence at the present time (Ball et al., 1995). News groups also allow for quick and easy browsing of the posted topics.

ACCESSING CLINICAL INFORMATION
FROM LIBRARIES

Nurse managers may need access to up-to-date clinical resources, information about issues and trends, current nursing management information, or other essential resources. Local libraries may not have extensive resources, or time may not be available to retrieve the materials from a library. The Internet can help access library information without the necessity of leaving the clinical area.

One Internet-accessible library is the Virginia Henderson International Nursing Library. This library maintains a collection of resources for Sigma Theta Tau International, including a collection of databases of timely information appropriate for nurses and administrators (Kirkpatrick & Kuipers, 1995). This library resource also contains material that may be difficult to obtain from traditional libraries, such as conference proceedings, unpublished nursing research, grant awards, and clinical protocols. In addition, the Henderson library contains researcher biographical data that may aid in networking with nursing researchers. By late 1994, this database contained 11,193 items, including the following: 4,042 demographic items, 4,601 projects, 581 dissertations, 717 conferences, 158 grants, 960 monographs, and 107 *Image* documents (Sigma Theta Tau International, 1996).

The Henderson library can be accessed on-line by using the Telnet command with the on-line address of <stti-sun.iupui.edu>. A free preview is available for visitors to the library. When requested to sign in at the library, use "visitor" for the user name and password. To enjoy full and unlimited access to the Henderson library, individuals can subscribe for $30 per year and libraries can subscribe for $90 per year.

Another available library resource is The Colorado Alliance of Research Libraries (CARL). The periodical database UnCover lists articles from more than 15,000 multidisciplinary journals (Nicoll, 1994c). CARL also provides the opportunity for direct distribution of articles, via FAX, for a small fee (usually around $10 per article). This service is advantageous if journals are not readily available. Use Telnet to access CARL at the address <pac.carl.org>. When requested to log in, type <pac>.

Another source of library-related materials of interest to nurse managers is the National Library of Medicine (NLM), part of the National Institute of

Health. NLM provides a wealth of health and medicine subscriptions, many of which are free. A good place to begin searching for medical-related information at the National Library of Medicine can be found at <nlm.nih.gov>. The NLM home page (http://www.nlm.nih.gov/) provides information about the library programs available and allows for connections to other NLM services. The NLM also has publications and software programs available via anonymous file transfer protocol (ftp://nlmpubs.nlm.nih.gov/). The NLM publications include materials such as AIDS information, fact sheets, and newsletters. Clinical practice guidelines are also available via the NLM (http://text.nlm.nih.gov/). Clinical specialty topics may also be available on-line (U.S. Department of Health and Human Services, 1995).

Other possible clinical-related sources of information are available on the Internet. Clinical information about breast cancer can be obtained through The Breast Cancer Information Clearinghouse (<nysernet.org>); information about maternal-child health topics is also available on-line (<mchnet.ichp.ufl.edu>). There are possibly thousands of other clinical resources available for nurses' use on the Internet (Tomaiuolo, 1995), and Table 4.3 provides some helpful WWW sites for getting started.

ON-LINE JOURNALS

The Internet is also experiencing growth of on-line journals. One example is the *OnLine Journal of Knowledge Synthesis for Nursing,* an electronic research journal that publishes clinically based research articles without the traditional lag time in publishing. The *OnLine Journal* subscription is $60 per year for individuals or $250 for libraries. A new on-line journal, *Online Journal of Issues in Nursing,* provides a forum for discussion on current issues related to clinical research, practice, and education. It is currently free of charge and accessible at the following address: <http://www.nursingworld.org/ojin/ohinhome.htm>.

Other health and related disciplines have electronic journals that may be relevant for nurses and managers. For example, *Mednews Health Infocom* newsletter is available by sending a subscription request via e-mail to <listserv@asuacad.bitnet>, or psychology information is available by subscribing to *Psychology* <listserv@pucc.bitnet> (Tomaiuolo, 1995).

Newsletters available through the World Wide Web also contain clinical information. Duke University publishes a newsletter accessible from their home page at URL <http://nursing-www.mc.duke.edu/nursing>. Other clinical agencies are beginning to include newsletter and patient care information on the Internet, such as the University of Iowa Hospitals and Clinics Publica-

TABLE 4.3 World Wide Web Sites

AACN (American Association of Critical-Care Nurses)
    http://www.aacn.org/
AMIA Nursing Work Group Home Page
    http://www.gl.umb.edu/~abbott/nurseinfo.html
American Journal of Nursing
    http://www.ajn.org/
American Nurses Association
    http://www.nursingworld.org/
Bo Graham Home Page
    http://vanbc.wimsey.com/_7Ebgraham/bo.html
Computers in Nursing Interactive
    http://www.cini.com/
Dee's Pain Management Page
    http://www.web-shack.com/dee/
Diane Wink's Home Page
    http://pegasus.cc.ucf.edu/~wink/home.html
NIGHTINGALE
    http://nightingale.con.utk.edu
Nursing and the NCLEX
    http://www.kaplan.com/nclex
Nursing Internet Resources
    http://medsrv2bham.ac.uk/nursing/resources/nurse-resources/
The "Virtual" Nursing Center
    http:www-sci.lib.uci.edu/HSG/Nursing.html
Virtual Hospital
    http://indy.radiology.uiowa.edu/VirtualHospital.html

---

tions <http://www.uihc.uiowa.edu/pubinfo/pubs.html>. These resources may be useful for nurse managers to share with the nursing staff, patients, or both.

FUNDING AND GRANT RESOURCES

The Internet can assist nurses in identifying funding and sources for special clinical projects. The National Institute of Health Guide to Grants and Contracts is available electronically by sending electronic mail subscription requests to <nihgde-L@jhuvm.hcf.jhu.edu>. Another grant source is the National Institutes of Health Grant Line, a bulletin board service that has information on public health service programs and policies (<wylbur. cu.nih.gov>) (Nicoll, 1994a).

MARKETING AND RECRUITMENT

As the health care industry becomes more competitive, institutions are marketing their services to attract the consumer dollar. Many agencies are using the Internet and WWW home pages for marketing and public relations purposes. Over one hundred hospitals now have links to MEDx, an Internet On-line Medical Exchange <http://www.medx.com/mxhospwl.html>. These hospitals range from 100-bed community hospitals to large tertiary medical centers in all states and around the globe. The HospitalWeb, a listing of hospital home pages, reports having more than 2,000 Internet users visiting the site in a month (Yerks, 1996). Nurse managers may want to view these hospital home pages to remain current with hospital trends nationwide. Nurse managers may also want to work with agency information specialists to showcase accomplishments that may attract potential employees or stimulate consumer business.

Another Internet use involves employment services; potential employees are using the Internet for job searching (Dutta, 1996). Nurse managers could use this service when looking for potential positions in management and executive areas. Recruiting agencies are now posting job information on the Web. One example of a growing list of recruiting agencies can be found on-line at <http://members.aol.com/TSBGeorge/>. Managers might use these employment services to recruit health care providers to their institution.

CONTINUING EDUCATION

Nurse managers and other health care providers may want access to continuing education programs for personal and professional growth. The Internet offers a variety of continuing education options, all of which are available 24 hours a day, 7 days a week. Universities are beginning to offer distance education through Internet communication (L. Nicoll, personal communication, 1996). The *American Journal of Nursing* has established a distance education project that offers continuing education course materials. These options are particularly attractive for nurse managers whose schedules may be incompatible with traditional offerings or for those in underserved areas of the country.

OTHER CONCERNS

As electronic communication continues to grow, users need to be aware of legal issues surrounding computer use. Confidentiality and privacy are not ensured with electronic mail. Others may have access to electronic mail messages, especially if using an employer's equipment. Messages sent or received may not be private, so careful consideration is essential when using electronic communication.

As World Wide Web materials are used, consideration must be given to copyright issues. Material available on the Internet may be copyrighted, so transfer and use of these files should comply with the copyright laws. It is illegal to distribute copyrighted material via electronic means unless granted permission (Edwards, 1995). Material utilized from the Internet should be appropriately referenced. An excellent reference for approved electronic resources is Li and Crane (1996).

CONCLUSION

Internet growth is exploding, and health care providers must keep up with the pace to provide appropriate and up-to-date care without relying solely on traditional computer record keeping. Valuable tools and new resources are being added to this growing global resource. This chapter provides an overview of capabilities available on the Internet, such as electronic mail, discussion and news groups, and information retrieval.

NOTE

It should be noted that every attempt to provide accurate information has been made; however, due to the dynamic nature and rapid growth of the Internet, changes occur frequently. Therefore, the addresses provided in this chapter may not be current at the time of publication. If an address provided is outdated, an Internet search using key terms may be conducted through a search engine such as Yahoo.

REFERENCES

Anderson, S. (1992). *Computer literacy for health care professionals.* New York: DelMar.

Ayre, R. (1995). Get connected: New paths to the net. *PC Magazine, 14*(17), 109-113.

Ball, M. J., Hannah, K. J., Newbold, S., & Douglas, J. V. (Eds.). (1995). *Nursing informatics: Where caring and technology meet.* New York: Springer.

DuBois, K., & Rizzolo, M. A. (1994). Cruising the "information superhighway." *American Journal of Nursing, 94*(12), 58-59.

Dutta, M. (1996, January 23). Internetworking. *Pittsburgh Post-Gazette,* pp. D-13, D-14.

Edwards, M. J. A. (1995). *The Internet for nurses and allied health professionals.* New York: Springer.

Gonzalez, E. L. F., & Seaton, H. J. (1995). Internet sources for nursing and allied health. *Database, 18*(3), 46-49.

Griffith, H. (1996). Internet magic. *Journal of Professional Nursing, 12*(1), 3.

Haynor, P. M., & Wells, R. M. (1992). Selecting a computerized staffing and scheduling system. In J. M. Arnold & G. A. Pearson (Eds.), *Computer applications in nursing education and practice* (pp. 147-155). New York: National League for Nursing.

Joos, I., Whitman, N. I., Smith, M. J., & Nelson, R. (1992). *Computers in small bytes.* New York: National League for Nursing.

Kehoe, B. P. (1994). *Zen and the art of the Internet.* Englewood Cliffs, NJ: Prentice Hall.

Kirkpatrick, J., & Kuipers, J. (1995). Negotiating two electronic resources for nursing. *Nursing Management, 26*(7), 68, 70, 72.

Lacefield, P. (1996, January 31). File: NRSINGED list. *Discussion List* [Online]. Available e-mail: NRSINGED@ulkyvm.bitnet [1996, January 31].

Levine, J. R., & Young, M. L. (1994). *Internet for dummies.* Foster City, CA: IDG Books.

Li, X., & Crane, N. B. (1996). *Electronic styles: A handbook for citing electronic information.* Medford, NJ: Information Today.

Marine, A., Kirkpatrick, S., Neou, V., & Ward, C. (1994). *Internet: Getting started.* Englewood Cliffs, NJ: Prentice Hall.

Nicoll, L. H. (1994a). Essential resources: On-line journals and magazines. *Journal of Nursing Administration, 24*(10), 14-16.

Nicoll, L. H. (1994b). An introduction to the Internet: Part I. History, structure, and access. *Journal of Nursing Administration, 24*(3), 9-11.

Nicoll, L. H. (1994c). An introduction to the Internet: Part II. Addresses and resources. *Journal of Nursing Administration, 24*(5), 11-13, 59.

Saba, V. K., Johnson, J. E., & Simpson, R. L. (1994). *Computers in nursing management.* Washington, DC: American Nurses Association.

Sigma Theta Tau International. (1996). *Electronic library* [On-line]. Available: Telnet stti-sun. iupui.edu

Simpson, R. L. (1995). "Surfing" the Internet. *Nursing Management, 26*(7), 18-19.

Tietze, M. R., & Huber, J. T. (1995). Electronic information retrieval in nursing. *Nursing Management, 26*(7), 36-42.

Tomaiuolo, N. G. (1995). Accessing nursing resources on the Internet. *Computers in Nursing, 13*(4), 159-164.

U.S. Department of Health and Human Services. (1995, March). *National Library of Medicine (NLM) Internet-accessible resources fact sheet.* Bethesda, MD: National Institutes of Health.

Wink, D. (1995). An introduction to nursing on the Internet. *Nurse Educator, 20*(6), 9-13.

Yerks, A. M. (1996). The Internet and pediatric nursing: Guide to the information superhighway. *Pediatric Nursing, 22*(1), 11-15.

CHAPTER 5

Computer Augmented Performance Evaluation

Cindy A. Scherb

Health care is experiencing tumultuous times. Investments in technology continue as human and financial resources decline. Financial hardships have created the need to downsize in organizations, along with an increased need to be more productive and to improve quality of patient care. A significant technological development has been computerized nursing information systems. Using computerized information can assist with improving nursing performance and the quality of patient care.

This chapter proposes an innovative management intervention: Computer Augmented Performance Evaluation. This intervention, which maximizes the decision support advantages fostered by integrating clinical and personnel systems, is not about designing a new performance evaluation form, but about enhancing the present evaluation system.

When performance evaluation is mentioned, everyone groans, managers and staff nurses alike. Nurse managers react negatively because they find evaluations time-consuming, subjective, and emotionally charged. They worry about being too nice or too harsh (Glover, 1989). If a manager is not familiar with the total work of the staff nurse, performance cannot be adequately evaluated (Gillies, 1994). For example, nurse managers may not be familiar with the work of staff nurses because they often do not work directly with the staff nurses on the same unit or because nurses may only work shifts when the nurse manager is not present.

Likewise, staff nurses react negatively to performance evaluations. They may view the evaluations as too subjective and pejorative. The nurse managers may be viewed as rating everyone as either high or low performers, rating nurses as the manager sees her- or himself, rating everyone in the middle, or viewing nurses' early behaviors as good or bad and continuing to rate all subsequent behavior in the same manner (Swansburg, 1996).

The goals of performance evaluations are to measure the achievement of nursing standards, reinforce nursing standards, and provide feedback to the employee (Fosbinder & Vos, 1989). The problems with evaluating performance as mentioned above have impeded the nursing profession's reaching these goals for decades. Many dollars and hours have been expended by organizations trying to develop performance evaluation systems that are meaningful and accurate. Despite these efforts, performance evaluation continues to be seen as a meaningless task by many nurse managers and staff nurses.

The purpose of this chapter is to propose an innovative management intervention, Computer Augmented Performance Evaluation, to be implemented with existing performance evaluations. Many nurses are unaware of the vast amount of data available through computerized systems. It may be known that the information is in the system, but not known if it is retrievable or in what form. This intervention is not about designing a new performance evaluation form, but offers ideas to enhance the present evaluation system by using data and information already available in clinical and personnel systems.

Computer augmented performance evaluation utilizes the information contained within computerized information systems to contribute more objective views of the nurses' performance, improve performance, and allow the evaluation process to be more continuous. This intervention not only supports auditing documentation, but also assists in defining nurse behavior.

SIGNIFICANCE AND RATIONALE
FOR THE INTERVENTION

Nursing management has an obligation to monitor professional nursing practice to assist the nursing staff to achieve quality patient care based on predetermined nursing standards. "The methods used to monitor professional nursing practice can be evaluative, developmental, and corrective in nature" (Smith, 1989, p. 7). Nurse managers need to use the information gathered to evaluate what the nurse has achieved, what has not been achieved, and what needs to be achieved in the future (Lunde & Durbin-Lafferty, 1986; Smith, 1989). Through the evaluation of job performance, multiple goals can be achieved, such as rewarding an excellent performer, enhancing performance through coaching, improving communication, and setting goals for the future (Gillies, 1994). Moreover, performance evaluations may provide valuable information to management about the effectiveness and efficiency of the management system (Megel, 1983). It is the monitoring of performance that enables quality patient care to be achieved.

"Performance evaluation is the measurement of the results of a person's work effort compared with previously agreed upon standards" (Ganong & Ganong, 1984, p. 60). Gillies (1994) states that an effective performance requires that the employee be familiar with the performance evaluation and the standards by which performance will be measured. Consequently, job descriptions and performance evaluation forms should be shared with the employee at orientation.

Evaluations of performance are not useful unless the supervisor completing the evaluation has adequate knowledge of the employee's behavior. If the supervisor does not have a representative sample of the nurse's performance, the evaluation may focus erroneously on either positive or negative behavior that may happen infrequently (Gillies, 1994).

An effective evaluation tool promotes objectivity, minimizes bias, and has reliability and validity. It is unlikely that bias can be completely removed from a tool nor that a tool will be totally objective. Bias can be controlled or minimized, however, by weighting certain items or limiting the number of items allowed on the tool not directly related to patient care, for example, grooming, dress. This strategy will prevent the nurse manager from placing too much focus on a single characteristic. Objectivity, the opposite of bias, requires that one remove oneself emotionally from a situation. Objectivity is enhanced when the focus of the evaluation is on role behaviors rather than personality traits (Gillies, 1994).

Because performance evaluations significantly impact future job performance (Gillies, 1994), it is important that evaluations have reliability and validity. Validity is established when the evaluation measures what it claims to measure. Reliability is exhibited when there is consistency in what the tool states it measures. This consistency can be obtained with comparison to other measures or by different evaluators arriving at the same conclusion about an employee's performance (Gillies, 1994; Megel, 1983).

Staff and supervisors need to be involved in the development and revision of performance evaluations (Nauright, 1987; Pelle & Greenhalgh, 1987). All criteria need to be understood to prevent confusion regarding the expected performance of an individual. Nurse managers and staff nurses need to be in agreement on the criteria selected and the standard level of performance required (Nauright, 1987).

Evaluation "is the process of appraising the meaning of data gathered through one or more measurements" (Litwack, Linc, & Bower, 1985, p. 5). These methods of measurement do not ensure the evaluation to be reliable and valid. The methods may be subjective in nature or limited in scope. By augmenting the evaluation process with a measure of performance through computerized information, an objective measure is added to the process.

With the widespread use of computerized documentation systems, a valuable avenue has been opened to collect data to enhance quality patient care and, at the same time, provide objective data for the evaluation process. The fact that computers can rapidly retrieve, summarize, and compare large volumes of information can facilitate the work of nurse managers in evaluating performance.

The Nursing Minimum Data Set (NMDS) is a database that can be used to advance nursing practice, improve patient care (Gallant, 1988), and enhance a performance evaluation system. These data can provide information on what types of patients are served by nursing, the reason they require nursing care, what care was provided, and the outcomes achieved from the health care system (Gallant, 1988). Another unique feature of the NMDS is the inclusion of the "unique number of principal registered nurse provider" (Werley, Ryan, Zorn, & Devine, 1994, p. 115). This unique number would identify clinicians across settings who are primarily responsible for a patient's care during a care episode. Although this identification system has not been developed, it could be designed around individual state licensure numbers (Werley & Lang, 1988). This system would allow patient data to be related to a particular nurse and retrieved as necessary.

At the present time, the NMDS as a whole is not widely used by hospitals. However, if the information contained within the NMDS on nursing diagnosis, interventions, outcomes, and intensity of nursing care (Werley & Lang, 1988) was captured in computerized nursing information systems, it would be possible to augment the evaluation process. A major roadblock to effective use of the NMDS is the lack of standardized language. Researchers in nursing continue to address this need for standardized language. The North American Nursing Diagnosis Association (NANDA) developed and continues to refine a taxonomy for standardizing nursing diagnoses (North American Nursing Diagnosis Association [NANDA], 1994). A classification of nursing interventions has been developed by the Iowa Intervention Project with the development of the Nursing Interventions Classification (NIC) taxonomy (Iowa Intervention Project, 1996). A taxonomy of nursing outcomes, The Nursing-Sensitive Outcomes Classification (NOC), has also been developed (Iowa Outcomes Project, 1997). These classification systems, and others, will greatly assist in standardizing nursing language and will enhance the process of capturing and retrieving relevant data from nursing information systems. In the meantime, even the nonstandardized nursing information stored within the computer systems can be of value for the evaluation process.

Although there is no research or literature on incorporating data obtained from nursing information systems into performance evaluation systems, there is a logical link between criteria on performance evaluations and data that are contained within most nursing information systems. Evaluations are based on a nurse's performance in direct and indirect patient care (Swansburg, 1996); performance can be evaluated, acknowledged, and enhanced through reviewing and utilizing computerized documentation.

POTENTIAL COMPUTERIZED VARIABLES

The computerized variables that could potentially be included in the computer augmented performance evaluation are outlined in Table 5.1. These variables will be discussed in greater length in the following section.

Most performance evaluations contain criteria related to the nurse's participation in care planning. The criteria may be a general criterion on care planning or a number of specific criteria related to *nursing diagnoses, interventions,* and *outcomes.* Computer information could enhance the performance evaluation by retrieving information for each nurse on the number of nursing diagnoses established, the most commonly established nursing diagnosis, the use of diagnoses specific to the unit or nursing standards, or combinations of these.

Clinical decision making can be evaluated through reviewing documentation of interventions. Information could be retrieved on interventions in the same manner as nursing diagnosis. One may be interested in knowing how many different interventions were utilized and/or what interventions were utilized with certain nursing diagnoses. Interventions can be reviewed and evaluated for appropriateness of choice and follow-up (Iowa Intervention Project, 1996). Samples of care plans could be retrieved to evaluate the appropriateness of interventions chosen for particular diagnoses.

At the present time, most outcomes are measured in some manner of being "met" or "not met." By retrieving this information from the computerized patient record, an evaluation could be completed as to the outcomes that a nurse, or the nursing staff as a whole, had achieved. If a unit had a system of nurse-patient accountability, such as primary nursing, outcome information would be very effective in evaluating a given nurse's performance.

Evaluation of completed care plans may be of interest to nurse managers and the nursing staff. A sample of care plans completed by a specific nurse could be

TABLE 5.1 Potential Computerized Variables

Nursing Diagnoses	Patient Satisfaction
Nursing Interventions	Employee Illness
Nursing Outcomes	Variance Tracking
Nurse-Patient Accountability	Continuing Education
Acuity	Professional Speaking
Medical Diagnosis	Professional Organizational Involvement
Indirect Nursing Interventions	Hospital Committee Involvement

obtained through the computer system and reviewed during the performance evaluation.

If a nursing unit has primary nursing or another system of *nurse-patient accountability*, a record could be retrieved as to the number of times a nurse was recorded as the primary nurse. In this time of downsizing and the increased use of nonprofessional assistive personnel, however, other patient care delivery systems will be utilized. In these delivery systems it will be harder to determine who is accountable for a given patient unless nursing devises a system of accountability. Such a system may entail assigning accountability based on who admits the patient, the number of days a nurse is assigned to care for a given patient, or possibly a case management system. Any of these systems would be useful in evaluating individual nurses' acceptance of accountability for specific patients. If the NMDS data elements were being collected, such evaluation could be accomplished through the linkage to an individual nurse caregiver provided by the unique RN provider number. In instances when this is not possible, the institution could collect this information by using the nurse's name or an institution-assigned unique identifier to be used for documentation purposes.

Almost all information systems contain patient classification or *acuity* information. Patient classification or acuity systems allow for grouping of patients according to the complexity and amount of nursing care required (Gillies, 1994). Although acuity information is most often used to determine staffing needs, it can also be useful in determining nursing performance. Acuity information could be aggregated for patients assigned to a particular nurse. This information would be useful in evaluating the level of patients that a given nurse cares for over a period of time. Insight could be gained as to the patient assignments a nurse is willing to handle or, indirectly, what level of patients co-workers, when making patient assignments, think a nurse can handle. This could be a measurement of growth of nursing ability over a period of time and an opportunity to reward performance or coach a nurse as necessary.

Medical diagnosis would provide information about the type of patients served on a given nursing unit and specifically by a particular nurse. A composite could be obtained exhibiting the types of patients cared for by a given nurse. This information would assist in evaluating the diversity of patients cared for by a nurse. A nurse could be recognized for developing expertise with a specialty patient population, or the composite may show a nurse lacks experience in caring for certain patient populations. If a nurse lacks experience in caring for certain patient populations, this information could be discussed at the evaluation and goals set to address the situation as appropriate.

The Nursing Interventions Classification (NIC) (Iowa Intervention Project, 1996) contains *indirect nursing interventions.* These interventions enhance patient care but are also important in determining staff participation in staff development of co-workers, professional development, and multidisciplinary involvement. Some of these interventions include Delegation, Preceptor: Employee, Preceptor: Student, Product Evaluation, Peer Review, Multidisciplinary Care Conference, and Research Data Collection. If utilizing NIC, documentation of these activities could be retrieved through the computerized system. If NIC is not a part of the documentation system, items such as these could be built into an information system. Reviewing documentation of these interventions would be an asset to the performance evaluation process.

Many hospitals gather *patient satisfaction* information by sending a questionnaire to the patient's home or by calling patients on the telephone after discharge. The information gathered is usually general in nature. The typical insights gleaned relate to environmental factors and maybe some comments regarding nursing. The comments concerning nursing are usually unspecified, but will occasionally include a positive or negative statement about a particular nurse, even if the nurse mentioned specifically by the patient may not have been the patient's primary nurse. By querying the computer system on the day of discharge, a list could be generated of three nurses who cared for the patient the most during the hospital stay and the patient's primary nurse, should the primary nurse not be one of the three names generated by the computer. The patient could then be asked, prior to discharge, to comment on the nursing care received from these nurses and nursing care received in general from the entire nursing staff.

The previous examples of retrievable variables have utilized the nursing information system as the source of data; however, all variables that could be included in a computer augmented performance evaluation are not contained within a nursing information system. The human resource and quality improvement departments may have databases that contain pertinent data for evaluating performance. Linkages, perhaps through a relational database, could be developed among the different systems, and information would be easily retrievable. The link among these systems could be a unique identifier number assigned to each nurse.

Linkage to human resource records would provide data of *employee illness.* These databases would be easy to query prior to evaluation to determine if this is an area to be addressed with the employee. The nurse manager would not need to rely on memory or to search through paper records containing the information in a nonsummarized form.

Likewise, the quality assurance department gathers data pertaining to quality improvement. *Variance reports* (e.g., variances on critical pathways, medication errors, etc.) would be one type of data collected by this department. Reviewing variance reports is usually a continuous process between the nurse manager and the staff. Variances are discussed as they occur. The yearly evaluation would be an excellent time to review, as a collective, all variances involving a particular nurse. It is easy to miss a trend that may be developing when reviewing the variances individually, but reviewing them once a year, collectively, can give insight to an area that may need improvement.

Professional development is often a portion of the performance evaluation, but information pertaining to professional development may be available only in written form. Participation in *continuing education, public speaking* activities at professional meetings and within the community, *membership in professional organizations,* and *committee involvement* with the organization are examples of professional development. This information could be computerized for ease of record keeping from year to year. Records could be maintained on an ongoing basis and data would be easily retrievable on a continuous basis and with performance evaluations.

Some of the information from computerized information systems has just been identified as possible criteria to supplement a performance evaluation system. This list is not exhaustive, but is a beginning format for any nurse manager and nursing staff.

The system should be designed so that the evaluation process is continuous instead of an annual event. One way to make the process continuous is to have the computerized data available to the nursing staff at any time between annual evaluations. Staff nurses should be able to access data upon which they are going to be evaluated and to compare themselves against the established standard. The staff nurse would then have the opportunity to change behavior to meet the standard if there is need for improvement.

Another important aspect of performance evaluations is the goal-setting process. Goal setting could still occur as an annual event, but by being able to access computerized data at any time, the nursing staff would be able to monitor their accomplishment of goals that they had identified for themselves.

The literature supports the need for objective, reliable, valid evaluation and performance feedback to the nursing staff. This management intervention attempts to identify appropriate computer data that can enhance the content and the process of performance evaluations.

EVALUATION

When introducing any intervention, it is important to measure whether the intervention was successful or not. There are four important outcomes for this intervention: (a) performance of staff nurses improves, (b) the staff perceive that the performance evaluation is more objective than it was previously, (c) retrieval of information regarding performance is easier, and (d) the evaluation process is more continuous. These outcomes need to be measured to assess if the desired effect was achieved. Other evaluation criteria may include cost of implementing and maintaining the system. The nurse manager and the nursing staff need to decide what measures will best show the effect of this intervention and to plan the collection of these measures at appropriate time frames within the intervention implementation.

SUMMARY

Health care is experiencing tumultuous times. Financial hardships have created the need to downsize in organizations, along with an increased need to be more productive and to improve quality of patient care. Advances in technology continue although human and financial resources shrink. Nursing has been impacted by all of these variables. The computerized nursing information system is a significant technological development that should be exploited to its full potential. Using computerized information can assist with enhancing nursing performance and improving the quality of patient care. A computer augmented performance evaluation may be one tool to achieve these objectives.

REFERENCES

Fosbinder, D., & Vos, H. (1989). Setting standards and evaluating nursing performance with a single tool. *Journal of Nursing Administration, 19*(10), 23-30.

Gallant, B. J. (1988). Data requirements for the Nursing Minimum Data Set as seen by a nurse administrator. In H. H. Werley & N. M. Lang (Eds.), *Identification of the Nursing Minimum Data Set* (pp. 165-176). New York: Springer.

Ganong, J. M., & Ganong, W. L. (1984). *Performance appraisal for productivity: The nurse manager's handbook.* Rockville, MD: Aspen Systems Corporation.

Gillies, D. A. (1994). *Nursing management: A systems approach.* Philadelphia: W. B. Saunders.

Glover, S. M. (Ed.). (1989). *Performance evaluations.* Baltimore, MD: Williams & Wilkens.

Iowa Intervention Project. (1996). In J. C. McCloskey & G. M. Bulechek (Eds.), *Nursing interventions classification (NIC)* (2nd ed.). St. Louis, MO: Mosby-Year Book.

Iowa Outcomes Project. (1997). In M. Johnson & M. Maas (Eds.), *Nursing outcomes classification (NOC).* St. Louis, MO: C. V. Mosby.

Litwack, L., Linc, L., & Bower, D. (1985). *Evaluation in nursing: Principles and practice.* New York: National League for Nursing.

Lunde, K. F., & Durbin-Lafferty, E. (1986). Evaluating clinical competency in nursing. *Nursing Management, 17*(8), 47-50.

Megel, M. A. (1983). Establishing a criterion-based performance appraisal for a department of nursing. *Nursing Clinics of North America, 18*(3), 449-456.

Nauright, L. P. (1987). Toward a comprehensive personnel system: Job description development: Part I. *Nursing Management, 18*(5), 54-56.

North American Nursing Diagnosis Association. (1994). *Nursing diagnosis: Definitions & classifications 1995-1996.* Philadelphia: Author.

Pelle, D., & Greenhalgh, L. (1987). Developing the performance appraisal system. *Nursing Management, 18*(12), 37-44.

Smith, T. C. (1989). A methodology to monitor professional nursing practice. *Journal of Nursing Quality Assurance, 3*(3), 7-23.

Swansburg, R. C. (1996). *Management and leadership for nurse managers* (2nd ed.). Sudbury, MA: Jones and Bartlett.

Werley, H. H., & Lang, N. M. (1988). The consensually derived Nursing Minimum Data Set: Elements and definitions. In H. H. Werley & N. M. Lang (Eds.), *Identification of the Nursing Minimum Data Set* (pp. 402-411). New York: Springer.

Werley, H. H., Ryan, P., Zorn, C. R., & Devine, E. C. (1994). Why the Nursing Minimum Data Set (NMDS)? In J. C. McCloskey & H. K. Grace (Eds.), *Current issues in nursing* (4th ed., pp. 113-122). St. Louis, MO: Mosby-Year Book.

CHAPTER 6

Nursing Information Systems: Administrative, Clinical, and Educational Applications

Sally Kellum
Mary Tatum

The purpose of this chapter is to discuss current innovations in information technology available to help nurse administrators cost-effectively meet the clinical, administrative, and educational needs of their service. The focus will be on three applications: clinical, staff development, and administrative applications.

National agencies, including the Joint Commission on Accreditation of Healthcare Organizations (JCAHO) and the Institute of Medicine (IOM), support nursing's participation in technology management and the vision of a computer-based patient record. The challenge facing nursing leaders is to ensure that innovative interactive systems are developed for all areas of nursing practice, including clinical, administrative, and educational. These systems must be critically evaluated to promote efficiency, productivity, and effectiveness in facilitating clinical decision making.

The integration of computer applications into health care has proven to be one of the most exciting technological advances in recent years. Its impact on nursing in particular has been dramatic. Computers are helping to improve the quality and efficiency of nursing care delivery through the use of information systems that facilitate the input, processing, and retrieval of patient information and nursing care planning programs that assist nurses with decision making.

Computer technology is evolving in health care and increasing its impact on nursing practice. Nurses use a computerized Hospital Information System more than any other group of heath care professionals (Hannah, Ball, & Edwards, 1994, p. vi). Computer technology has improved task performance in administration, clinical practice, research, and education areas. Emerging from this technology is an innovative role for nurses. The role of the informatics nurse is to "analyze, design, develop, modify, implement, evaluate, or maintain information handling technologies that collect patient and client data to support the practice of nursing" (American Nurses Association, 1995, p. iii). Information-handling technologies exist to support clinical practice, staff development, and administration.

APPLICATION OF COMPUTER
TECHNOLOGY IN CLINICAL PRACTICE

The application of computer technology in clinical practice is an area that nursing needs to embrace in order to capture patient data and decrease redundant documentation. Computers are used to facilitate accuracy and speed in diagnosis and treatment.

In addition to the use of computers for medical imaging and laboratory analysis, computer systems have also been developed to serve interpretive functions. As described by Bronzino (1982), these systems can enhance care by facilitating the accuracy of results and diagnosis and by returning the results with great rapidity. For example, EKG and pulmonary function test interpretation can be accomplished with systems dedicated to these specific functions. A critical component of these applications is that they need to communicate with the hospital information system (HIS). A basic component of a hospital information system is a design for the maintenance of patients' records in a consistent fashion. Patient information can be stored in the system and retrieved as necessary. The CEO of the Medical Center of Delaware stated that the difference between a health care delivery system and an integrated health care delivery system is the capability for a patient to enter the system at any point of service and have all necessary and appropriate information available to the caregiver (Keever, 1995).

AUTHORS' NOTE: The information in this chapter is the opinions of the authors and does not necessarily reflect the opinion of the Department of Veterans Affairs.

Radiology

Computers are frequently used for medical imaging (CAT scans, MR imaging, ultrasound). The most recent development is a technology called computed radiography. This technology promises to convert all general radiological films to an electronic form. Radiology would become a filmless process and allow multiple users to view the results on workstations in different areas of a hospital and even at remote sites such as a physician's office, rural hospital, or clinic. "Integration of computer-driven information systems is now recognized as a general need of medical practice. The 'filmless' hospital has been demonstrated as a model for the future" in the Department of Defense and at the Baltimore, Maryland, VA Medical Center (Shannon, 1995, p. 295).

Laboratory

Computers have also made laboratory analysis of specimens more accurate, efficient, and objective. In today's environment of managed care and cost consciousness, many laboratories are negotiating outreach programs. As a by-product of these affiliations, each facility will need to be networked through the hospital information system to enhance the ordering and receiving of results. A mobile lab may work with another facility to complete laboratory analysis. A standardized vocabulary and policies to disseminate results electronically are required when working with multiple sites.

Computerized Patient Care Record

With a hospital information system (HIS), patient records are more complete (Rosenberg, Glueck, Stroebel, Reznikoff, & Ericson, 1969), accessible (Lincoln & Korpman, 1980), and legible (Greene, Kerr, Likely, & Stephenson, 1982) than those that are handwritten and manually accessed. Thus, quality and accuracy of documentation are improved, and information is easily transferred from department to department, increasing the efficiency of communication (Staggers, 1988). Advantages for nursing include time savings through reducing clerical activities, elimination of duplicate effort, and more effective use of personnel (Hannah et al., 1994). A computerized patient record system can provide the health care provider with better practice management, integrated accounting systems for office or clinic, the ability to link inpatient and outpatient records, and a problem-oriented display of the patient record (Ball & Collen, 1992). Overall, an HIS increases productivity, decreases time on tasks, and is cost-effective, often resulting in labor reductions (Blask, Cleary, & Dux, 1985).

A number of ethical and legal issues have emerged as a result of HISs. Ensuring the confidentiality of computerized patient information has become a major focus (Albarado, McCall, & Thrane, 1990; Frawley, 1995). Individual patient records should be inaccessible to "unauthorized" personnel, that is, anyone not directly responsible for that person's care. Generally, this can be accomplished by assigning authorized users specific access codes or passwords. In many cases, these codes can be used to access only certain kinds of data from terminals at specific locations.

In health care informatics today there is a lot of discussion and emphasis on developing the computer-based patient record (CPR). The Institute of Medicine (IOM) has set "Gold Standard" criteria that are shaping the CPR. The 12 attributes that all vendors and institutions are attempting to achieve are as follows:

- Provide a problem list
- Measure health status (especially in terms of outcome-based patient care)
- Document clinical reasoning
- Provide linkages (longitudinal records within a system as well as linking to other systems)
- Protect against unauthorized access
- Support continuous access
- Support simultaneous multiuser views
- Support other clinical resources
- Facilitate clinical problem solving
- Support direct data entry by physicians
- Support management of patient care
- Provide flexibility and expansibility

The CPR system should be the engine that enables an organization's ability to perform outcomes and quality studies and to feed that data directly back to the care process at the point of care (Dick & Andrew, 1996). At the Veterans Affairs Medical Center in Durham, an unpublished project demonstrated that giving the provider feedback on patterns of laboratory test ordering increased the appropriateness of lab test orders and decreased redundancy, thereby reducing cost, when compared to a control group that was not given feedback. This was a Duke University Chief Resident Project, and the primary author was Kurt Bodily, MD.

The VA's version of the CPR system is called Computerized Patient Record System (CPRS). Version 1.0, released in October 1996, integrates and enhances many of the clinical applications currently found in the Decentralized Hospital Computer Program (DHCP) hospital information system and can operate under a graphical user or terminal interface (see Table 6.1). CPRS Version 1.0

demonstrates clear progression toward the goal of achieving all of the IOM's Gold Standard attributes of a computer-based patient record. When considering a CPRS, the following components and systems warrant close examination: point-of-care technology, patient data management systems, physician order entry, and nursing systems.

Point of Care. Many facilities are implementing wireless systems that provide connection via airwaves to the NIS (Nursing Information System) or HIS. These systems resemble laptop computers and are being used on rounds for entering orders while seeing the patient. The current trend is for the computer devices to be portable so that data can be entered at the "point of care." The initial response to this type of system has been very positive: The computer moves with the practitioner, eliminating the need for notes and then transcription of that data into the terminal (Figure 6.1). In the Veterans Affairs Medical Center in Durham, North Carolina, bedside terminals are mounted on a rolling device in the critical care areas. These terminals can be raised for standing or lowered for use from a chair. These terminals are also attached to a long cord that allows the device to be moved outside the patient's room for privacy or for isolation cases (see Figures 6.2 and 6.3).

Patient Data Management Systems. The management of high-volume clinical information, such as that commonly obtained on patients in critical care settings, can also be facilitated with the use of information systems dedicated solely to this function. Patient Data Management Systems (PDMS) have emerged in critical care settings. These more advanced systems utilize computerized patient monitoring and also allow for the storage and integration of data from these systems. In these areas, the hemodynamic information displayed on the bedside monitor and ventilators is directly entered into the computerized patient chart. It is the role of the nurse and respiratory therapist to verify the accuracy of the data prior to storing. Data can also be manually entered (e.g., patient assessments, care plans, treatment records) or made available to the system through linkage with other parts of the hospital information system (e.g., the laboratory).

One of the challenges facilities face is working with vendors to integrate vendors' systems with the hospital information system. Presently, the only links with the Hewlett Packard CareVue system are with lab data and ventilator data. The system has the ability to document patient data (flowsheet), progress notes, care plans, and medication administration. Each of these applications is a separate screen in the computer; they do not communicate with each other. This product allows the hospital to customize the documentation tools and

TABLE 6.1 Computerized Patient Record System (CPRS)

Computerized Patient Record System- (CPRSGUI)	A graphical user interface ("Windows"-type environment) that provides a comprehensive presentation of the patient record.
CPRS-List Manager	The List Manager Interface provides a comprehensive presentation of the patient record for the CRT ("dumb terminal") user.

Supporting Module	Description
Order Entry	Provides event-driven, standardized ordering capabilities for physicians, nurses, and other hospital personnel.
Notifications	Provides a clinical alerting system that notifies providers of significant patient care issues in an event-driven environment.
Order Check Expert System	Created for the CPRS to display event-driven alerts for providers during the ordering process to conditions that may contraindicate the order.
Radiology/Nuclear Medicine	Includes additional functionality for radiology as well as extensive modifications to receive, process, and provide status updates for radiology orders from Order Entry in an event-driven environment.
Laboratory Inpatient Pharmacy Outpatient Pharmacy Adverse Reaction Tracking Dietetics	Receives, processes, and provides status updates for orders from Order Entry in an event-driven environment. These packages also provide information for display on the CPRS.
Patient Information Management System (PIMS)	Supports patient movement events and update of patient-provider linkages in the CPRS in an event-driven environment.
Vitals	Provides vital signs information for display in the CPRS.
Consults Tracking	Receives, processes, and provides status updates for consult orders from Order Entry in an event-driven environment. It also provides information for display in the CPRS.
Text Integration Utility (TIU)	Standardizes document handling in DHCP. In addition to operating as a stand-alone application to support Progress Notes, Discharge Summary, and History and Physical-type documents, TIU will receive and process clinical documents in an event-driven environment within the CPRS and provide information for display.
Authorization/ Subscription Utility (ASU)	Allows sites to associate users with user classes, allowing them to specify the level of authorization needed to sign or order specific document types and orderables. It is designed to eventually support all applications, providing a means for Medical Centers to manage electronic signature and notification requirements.
Patient Care Management Module (PCMM)	Provides team and personal list functionality for the CPRS in an event-driven environment.
Patient Postings	A component developed as part of the TIU, Patient Postings provides a mechanism for posting pertinent patient information in the CPRS (e.g., "Patient can be violent").

(Continued)

TABLE 6.1   Continued

Supporting Module	Description
Imaging	Provides imaging capabilities for display in a "Windows"-type environment.
Problem List	Receives and processes patient problem data from the CPRS and other Data Capture methods and will provide information for display. Problem List allows linkage to associated clinical data, such as medication and exams.
Automated Information Capture System	Allows clinicians and others to create on-line encounter forms that provide lists of information for patient management as well as for display in CPRS to facilitate capture of the Ambulatory Care Minimum Data Set.
Lexicon Utility	Provides standardized vocabulary for the capture of procedures and diagnoses within the CPRS; is also available for other applications to use.
Scheduling	Provides linkage between orders and patient appointments in the CPRS in an event-driven environment.
Patient Care Encounter	Acts as a data repository for clinical information entered through many data capture methods, including electronic scanners and the CPRS; information stored in PCE can be displayed on Health Summaries or other reports or in the CPRS.
Visit Tracking	Provides visit orientation for clinical data entered through CPRS as well as for other DHCP applications.

SOURCE: Adapted from Andrus, 1996.

provides a quick response time to trouble calls. A paramount concept that each facility must keep in mind is that it will need to grow with a vendor toward future applications and integration.

The PDMS used at the Veterans Affairs Medical Center in Durham can trend and analyze dysrhythmias. Monitors alarm once preset parameters are violated. In the coronary care unit, a system continuously analyzes 12-lead EKGs and alarms when there is evidence of cardiac ischemia. This system also trends minute-to-minute EKG and pressure waveform data capture. This feature is very useful in reviewing events after an arrest or for trends in cardiac rhythm patterns. Inherent in the critical care documentation system are a variety of calculations, including those used to determine optimal drug dosages and administration intervals in selected situations. Today, more and more patient data management systems are being linked to either an NIS or an HIS. For PDMS to keep pace with the rapid change in information technology, they must be fully incorporate their system into the HIS.

Physician Order Entry. In actuality, there are two subsets to an order entry system: the order entry component and the results reporting component. The

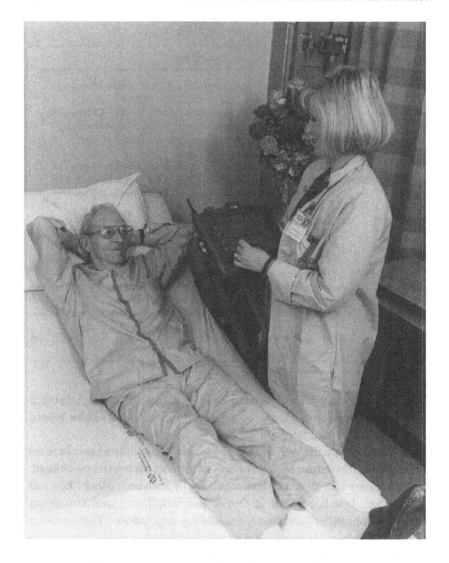

Figure 6.1. Health care provider using hand-held point-of-care device.
SOURCE: Photo copyright by Telxon Corporation. Used with permission.

order entry system should allow physician or nurse order entry from all areas
of the hospital (Ball, Hannah, Jelger, & Peterson, 1988). This requires installation of terminals in all nursing units, patient care areas, and ancillary departments, as well as availability of modem dial-in from remote locations. Order

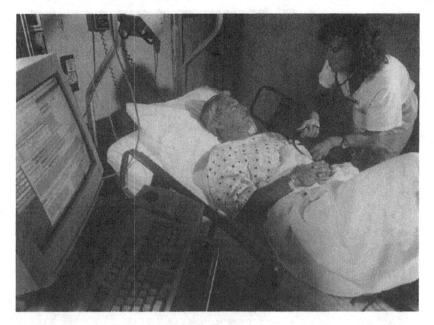

Figure 6.2. Nurse at bedside, using bedside terminal.
SOURCE: Photo copyright Hewlett Packard Company. Used with permission.

entry systems provide an efficient method for clinicians to enter all patient orders and for displaying results of patient orders.

In the Durham Department of Veterans Affairs Medical Center, physicians have begun directly entering their orders into the hospital information system. With direct entry of orders, there is a marked decrease in medication errors; transcription errors are almost totally eliminated. The use of this system has improved the legibility and efficiency of orders as well as assisted in retrieval of information on ordering trends for analysis. Clinicians seeing the patient for the first time are able to generate data displaying all the current medications and any adverse reactions there might have been to medications or food products. The pharmacy component within the order entry system generates a laser printed medication administration record for nurses to use in administering medications. At other VA facilities, nurses utilize wireless systems for electronically documenting the administration of medications.

Nursing Systems. According to the Center for Healthcare Information Management's (CHIMS) *Nurse Executive's Guide to Directing and Managing Nurse*

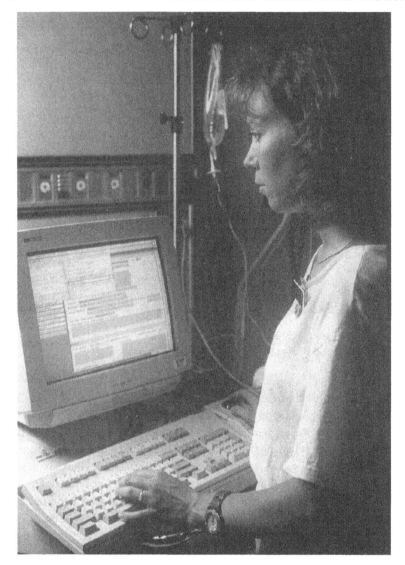

Figure 6.3. Nurse entering data into bedside terminal.
SOURCE: Photo copyright Hewlett Packard Company. Used with permission.

Information Systems, a nursing information system (NIS) is a software system that automates the nursing process from assessment to evaluation, including patient care documentation. It also includes a means to manage the data necessary for the delivery of patient care (i.e., patient classification, staffing, scheduling, and costs). An effective NIS cannot live in isolation, but must be an integral component of a larger clinical information system–along with physician and other caregiver components (Hughes & Andrew, 1995). This integration becomes crucial as patient care delivery and documentation become more interdisciplinary.

The VA Hospital Information Software includes modules for documenting Progress Notes, Nursing/Patient Care Planning, Vital Signs, and Intake and Output (which includes documentation for assessment of IV sites). The care planning module contains model standard care plans and can generate patient care plans including information on patient problems, goals, outcomes, interventions/orders, dates of problem evaluation/resolution, target dates for accomplishing goals, and related risk factors. These care plans can be customized for individual patients or to support Standards of Patient Care as identified at each VA facility (Medical IRM Office, 1995). The Care Plan application also produces patient assignment worksheets that include patient problems, nursing orders, and information from the Order Entry package. There is also a software application called Health Summary that allows the user to customize patient information. Some of the templates used today include data such as active medications, laboratory tests, clinic visits and progress notes, allergies, problem lists, discharge summaries, and the presence of an advanced directive. These data, displayed within 1 or 2 minutes, can be printed when individuals want to look at the information in a written format. The individual user can request historical data for various time frames. These data can be accessed from any terminal within the facility as well as remotely. This software is utilized by physicians, nurse practitioners, and physician assistants, as well as nursing staff. The weakest link in the nursing documentation system is the Progress Notes package, currently a free text application. Free text entry of computer documentation does not lend itself to data retrieval, and therefore does not provide any benefit for administrators in terms of decision support or data analysis. In early 1997, the Progress Notes and Discharge Summaries packages were integrated into the Text Integration Utilities package, standardizing document handling.

APPLICATION OF COMPUTER
TECHNOLOGY IN STAFF DEVELOPMENT

The introduction of computer technology has had a tremendous impact on the teaching/learning process. Computer-assisted instruction (CAI) materials are being used more and more frequently for the education of nurses in a variety of clinical settings. For orientees in the health professions, CAI can be used as the main or an alternate teaching strategy to assist nurses in mastering course content. Use of CAI can be a required activity or recommended for extra guidance or remediation. For staff nurses, CAI provides opportunity for continuing education.

CAI programs include games, tutorials, drill and practice programs, and simulations. Simulations allow users to apply knowledge of some content area in a simulated "real-life" situation described on a computer screen; decision-making abilities can be tested with the use of this type of CAI. Many CAI programs integrate tutorial, drill and practice, and simulation components in one software program. At the Durham VA, the use of CAI has facilitated the teaching of medication calculations in the medical surgical areas and recognizing dysrhythmias in the critical care areas and emergency care areas.

Interactive video systems integrate the use of video and computer-assisted-learning in an automatic, interactive fashion. The combination of video and CAI make learning even more stimulating and realistic. At the Durham VA, advanced cardiac life support instruction can be accomplished using the American Heart Association CPR/ACLS Learning System, which simulates medical emergencies and utilizes sensorized manikins to determine if compression, inflation, and intubation techniques performed by the user are correct. This technology is also being used to validate competencies for respiratory therapists on intubation techniques. Over a 2-year period, 42 nursing staff completed the criteria for ACLS. The range in time for course completion was from 3 to 12 hours, with the average of 6 hours regardless of whether it was revalidation or an initial exposure to ACLS (see Figure 6.4).

Traditional ACLS courses require a minimum of 16 hours training time per individual at a tuition cost of $125. Assuming an average RN salary of $22/hour, the total salary cost per participant is $352 and the total ACLS cost (tuition and salary) is $477. Over a 2-year period, 36 nurses completed the 2-day course and six nurses completed a 1-day revalidation. If traditional teaching methods had been used, 624 hours of training time would have been required. The tuition cost would have been $4,500 for the 2-day classes and $450 for the revalidation course. Using the American Heart Association CPR/ACLS Learning System, the 42 nurses used only 272 hours for training, saving 352 training hours ($7,744), which were redirected into patient care activities (see Table 6.2). Over a 2-year period, the final benefits of using this technology included a combined salary and tuition cost avoidance of $12,694; an increased percentage of ICU nurses having completed the ACLS course criteria (increased from 10% [8 persons] to 64% [50 persons]); and an overall reduced anxiety during ACLS completion (see Figure 6.5).

When compared with lecture as a teaching strategy, CAI has been proven to be at least as effective as lecture (Gaston, 1988). Computer-assisted-learning

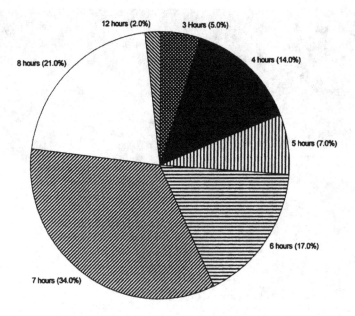

Figure 6.4. Time to complete computerized ACLS.

Table 6.2 Cost of Traditional ACLS Compared to AHA CPR/ACLS System

Method of Teaching	No. Nurses	Tuition ($)	No. Hrs	Salary Cost ($)	Total Cost ($)	Total Cost Avoidance ($)
Traditional ACLS						
New Course Completion	36	4,500	576	12,672	17,172	18,678
Revalidation	6	450	48	1,056	1,506	– 5,984
AHA CPR/ACLS System	42	n/a	272	5,984	5,984	12,694

provides a self-directed and cost-effective means of education that is an alternative or adjunct to traditional teaching methods. These educational methods have been found to be most effective when used in combination with other learning experiences. Many programs maintain records of each user's performance, providing documentation of teaching/learning activities for legal, continuing education, and/or accreditation purposes. Well-developed CAI/IVD programs utilize colorful and graphical designs; provide prompt feedback regarding correct and incorrect decisions; and are easy to use with very few keystrokes.

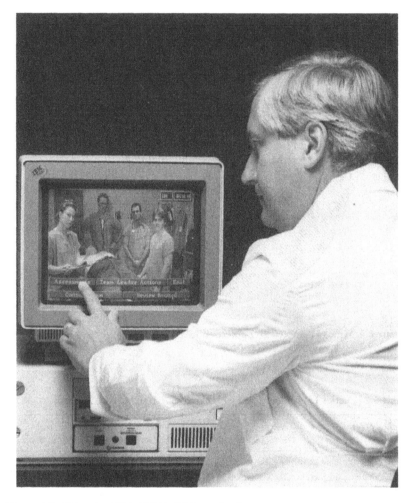

Figure 6.5. Using the AHA CPR/ACLS Learning System.
SOURCE: Photo copyright by American Heart Association CPR/ACLS Learning System.

APPLICATION OF COMPUTER
TECHNOLOGY IN ADMINISTRATION

The availability and management of data for decision making are critical for nurse administrators. Administrative applications, consisting of patient classification (acuity) systems for inpatient areas, were the core components of early nursing information systems (NIS). Administrative applications can be classified in two ways (Hannah et al., 1994): those that provide nurse managers with information for decision making, or "management information systems"; and those that help nurse managers in communicating decisions, also called "nursing office automation systems."

Nursing management information systems include systems for patient classification, nursing workload, and unit staffing as well as human resource management. The Durham VA facility's nursing information system allows classification of patients and provides acuity data for medical, surgical, nursing home, intensive care, psychiatry, hemodialysis, and recovery room areas. Other VA facilities also utilize classification systems for intermediate care, spinal cord injury, domiciliary, and substance abuse patients. Classification systems provide a measurement of nursing intensity. These patient-specific data facilitate analysis of workload trends and assist managers in the allocation of resources, both daily and long term. Nurse administrators, however, must critically evaluate their classification systems for validity and reliability as well as continually monitor the interrater reliability of classification systems among the clinical areas. Future directions for patient classification will include expansion of classification systems or workload management systems for ambulatory and home care settings. As much of the health care shifts from inpatient areas to ambulatory care and home settings, nurse administrators are challenged to identify workload and to analyze trends across all settings in which nursing care is delivered.

Staff record tracking is another core administrative function utilized. This application tracks data on nursing employee demographics, position control, salary and job classification, personnel information, professional education and skills, licensure, professional certification and dates for recertification, professional experience (which also documents career paths), as well as dates of annual performance evaluations and promotions. The staff tracking function also tracks annual inservice education sessions and continuing education.

The VA hospital information system does not include a Nurse Scheduler, although many facilities utilize commercial schedulers that integrate with the hospital information system. Nurses enter clinical manhours worked on each unit each shift by category (RN, LPN, NA). These data are compared to the classification data for each unit to generate unit and service level Workload Statistics reports. The hospital information system, while lacking a scheduling system, does have a payroll system that tracks employee time and attendance. All time worked is certified by the nurse manager biweekly. The system allows for tracking of vacation time, holidays, and sick time records for each employee, as well as overtime and compensatory time used.

Nursing office automation systems include software tools that assist nurse administrators and other nursing staff in communication. These systems include electronic mail, voice mail, and word processing and spreadsheet application software. At the Durham VA facility, each nurse manager has a personal computer in his or her office that includes access to the hospital information system as well as electronic mail, Microsoft Word, and Microsoft Excel. These tools assist the nurse manager in maintaining accountability for the human, fiscal, and physical resources on his or her unit. All nursing service employees have access to and are oriented to the electronic mail system, and mailgroups have been set up within the Nursing Department for nursing units and job category (e.g., "RN," "LPN," "NA," "Nurse Managers," etc.), as well as for committees and task forces within the Nursing Department and interdisciplinary groups throughout the Medical Center. Electronic mail facilitates rapid communication and minimizes the generation of paper for communication.

Integral to health care information systems of the future will be systems that assist clinicians in making clinical decisions with regard to patient care. Such a system is called a decision support system (DSS). A decision support system for nursing serves as a computerized consultant; it provides a comprehensive database of information and advice regarding the care of patients with specific health problems (Brennan, 1988). A decision support system can be designed utilizing artificial intelligence techniques (a branch of computer science that uses logic), in which the knowledge and logical thinking of a domain expert is encoded into a computer program. The result is called an expert system (Brennan, 1988). The focus in most expert systems in nursing has been nursing diagnoses, care planning, and patient assessment. Decision support systems are presently being used in several facilities across the country. In these cases the decision support system is integrated in the HIS, providing both financial analysis and clinical analysis.

An example of a decision support system function utilizing programmed logical thinking of a domain expert is real-time tracking of critical pathways. Through this tracking, case managers can be notified through the computer when a patient has experienced a predetermined "critical event" that would require an immediate case review. These systems are dependent on computerized documentation. As all disciplines document via the computer, the true potential will be fulfilled with real-time analysis and synthesis of patient data.

Decision support systems provide data on patterns of care and patient outcomes linked to resource consumption and costs associated with the health care processes. The VA DSS is a secondary relational database that integrates selected elements from each patient's resource utilization and clinical outcomes to permit evaluation of patterns of care for given patient populations (DSS Program Office, 1995). The decision support system database is extracted from existing VA clinical and administrative data systems. The functional capabilities of decision support systems (DSS Program Office, 1995) include

- Budgeting and planning for medical centers based on case-specific workload
- Resource distribution to the medical centers based on performance
- Support of managed care for the VHA System
- Equitable comparison of Medical Centers
- Support of Quality Management
- Productivity analysis and patient specific costs

Initiatives for cost reduction and managed competition create new demands for decision support (Ball, Simborg, Albright, & Douglas, 1995). The ability to integrate information about patterns of patient care outcomes with resource utilization provides administrators with insight about the value of health care services at their facility and allows comparison (benchmarking) with other facilities. This knowledge is critical for the VA's growth and survival in a competitive health care environment (DSS Program Office, 1995). Implementation of DSS throughout the entire VA system is occurring over a 39-month period. In addition to facilitating resource management decision making, DSS also allows managers to focus on opportunities to improve clinical practice patterns.

CONCLUSION/SUMMARY

This is an era in which many innovations exist in information technology. A comprehensive clinical information system should involve processes that do not "duplicate" the paper record, but redefine and streamline the processes involved in patient care. The future computerized patient record will consist of a computerized chart that has critical information, and that follows the patient through all care encounters.

With decreasing resources in staff development departments, there is a need to look for creative teaching strategies to increase learning and decrease lecture times. Advantages of quality computer-assisted instruction and interactive video include ensured consistency of presentation; provision of caregiving experiences in a protected environment; self-paced, effective, and enjoyable teaching-learning strategy; increased retention; reduction in educator time; and cost savings.

In this era of managed care and cost containment, administrative applications are assisting nurse administrators to take a more active role in the financial management of their work environments. Nurse managers and administrators need appropriate data available at their fingertips. The ability of computers to retrieve, summarize, and compare information rapidly has proven very useful for nurse administrators; unfortunately, only a few hospitals have integrated hospital information systems that allow for concurrent on-line data retrieval (Hannah et al., 1994). Integrated systems are crucial to efficient functioning. Data should be entered in the system only once and should be available wherever needed. Systems must be critically evaluated to promote efficiency, productivity, and effectiveness in facilitating clinical and administrative decision making. Future hospital information systems must also be able to support intraorganizational integration and interorganizational networking.

The challenge for nurse administrators and informatics nurses is to ensure that hospital information systems provide clinicians with the information necessary to manage patient care and provide managers information necessary for managing patient care units within the organization, such as resource allocation and utilization, personnel management, planning and policy making, and decision support (Hannah et al., 1994). Innovative, interactive systems need to be developed for all areas of nursing practice: clinical, administrative, and educational. Nurse administrators must be able to identify organizationwide and nursing-specific information and technology needs as well as to organize, coordinate, and develop information system management (Ball et al., 1995).

REFERENCES

Albarado, R. S., McCall, V., & Thrane, J. M. (1990). Computerized nursing documentation. *Nursing Management, 21*(7), 64-65.

American Nurses Association. (1995). *Standards of practice for nursing informatics.* Washington, DC: American Nurses Publishing.

Andrus, R. (1996). *CPRS and supporting modules* (unpublished table). Salt Lake City, UT: VA Medical Information Resource Management Field Office.

Ball, M. J., & Collen, M. F. (Eds.). (1992). *Aspects of the Computer-based Patient Record.* New York: Springer.

Ball, M. J., Hannah, K. J., Jelger, G. U., & Peterson, H. (Eds.). (1988). *Nursing informatics: Where caring and technology meet.* New York: Springer.

Ball, M. J., Simborg, D. W., Albright, J. W., & Douglas, J. V. (Eds.). (1995). *Healthcare information management systems: A practical guide* (2nd ed.). New York: Springer.

Blask, D., Cleary, J., & Dux, L. (1985, December). A computerized medical information system— Sustaining benefits previously achieved. *Health Care and Computers,* pp. 60-64.

Brennan, P. (1988). DSS, ES, AI: The lexicon of decision support. *Nursing and Health Care, 9*(9), 501-503.

Bronzino, J. D. (1982). *Computer applications for patient care.* Menlo Park, CA: Addison-Wesley.

Decision Support System Program Office. (1995). *Decision support system: Executive briefing.* Bedford, MA: Department of Veterans Affairs, Veterans Health Administration.

Dick, R., & Andrew, W. (1996). The CPR: An evaluative perspective. *Healthcare Informatics, 13*(2), 104-106.

Frawley, K. (1995). Achieving the CPR while keeping an ancient oath. *Healthcare Informatics, 12*(4), 28-30.

Gaston, S. (1988). Knowledge, retention, and attitude effects of computer-assisted instruction. *Journal of Nursing Education, 27*(1), 30-34.

Greene, R., Kerr, H., Likely, N., & Stephenson, P. (1982). Computers and patients: The user system. *Canadian Nurse, 78*(9), 34-36.

Hannah, K. J., Ball, M. J., & Edwards, M. J. (1994). *Introduction to nursing informatics.* New York: Springer.

Hughes, S., & Andrew, W. (1995). Automating nursing from assessment to evaluation. *Healthcare Informatics, 12*(4), 36-50.

Keever, G. W. (1995). Integrated delivery systems: Virtuality becomes reality. *Healthcare Informatics, 12*(10), 47-50.

Lincoln, T. L., & Korpman, R. A. (1980). Computers, health care, and medical information science. *Science, 210,* 257-263.

Medical IRM Office. (1995). *Decentralized hospital computer program.* Birmingham, AL: Department of Veterans Affairs, Medical Information Resources Management Office.

Rosenberg, M., Glueck, B. C., Jr., Stroebel, C. F., Reznikoff, M., & Ericson, R. P. (1969). Comparison of automated nursing notes as recorded by psychiatrists and nursing service personnel. *Nursing Research, 18*(4), 350-357.

Shannon, R. H. (1995). Computer-enhanced radiology: A transformation to imaging. *Healthcare information management systems: A practical guide* (pp. 283-296). New York: Springer.

Staggers, N. (1988). Using computers in nursing. *Computers in Nursing, 6*(4), 164-169.

CHAPTER 7

Accessibility to Knowledge for Research-Based Practice

Carol L. Ireson
Cathie L. Velotta

A 10- to 15-year gap exists between the development of research-based knowledge and its use in practice. Accessibility to knowledge can narrow the gap. In this chapter, the authors describe a strategy developed to increase nurses' accessibility to research-based knowledge via the computer and evaluate the extent of its success. Adoption of innovations such as this can be facilitated when diffusion theory is used to guide the change process.

As a result of the technology explosion in health care, patients must undergo hundreds of different diagnostic tests and procedures. These procedures cause patients to experience anxiety that can extend their recovery period. Concrete, objective information has been demonstrated to have a positive effect on a patient's response to stressful diagnostic and treatment experiences. Knowledge about this process has been developing since the early 1970s, when Jean Johnson (1974) published her seminal work on the effect of accurate expectations on reactions to noxious medical exams. Christman, Kirchhoff, and Oakley (1992) recommended that the preparation for patients undergoing anxiety-producing procedures should include information about sensations they commonly experience. Despite this knowledge, nurses do not consistently use this sensory information in preparing patients for stressful diagnostic events.

BACKGROUND

Knowledge Utilization and Diffusion Theory

Promoting the utilization of research-based knowledge by nurses within the practice setting continues to be a challenge for the nursing discipline. Bostrom and Wise (1994) suggested that a 10- to 15-year gap exists between the generation of research-based innovations and the application of these innovations in practice. An *innovation* is defined as any idea, practice, or objective perceived as new by an individual, a group, or an organization (Rogers, 1983). Pettengill, Gillies, and Clark (1994) compared the research utilization process to the innovation diffusion process described by Rogers (1983). The extent of nurses' adoption of an innovation has been measured using the stages from the innovation-decision process: awareness of the idea, persuasion, decision about using the idea, the actual implementation of the idea, and confirmation with others. Studies of nurses' adoption of research findings revealed that nurses had moved beyond the stage of awareness to that of persuasion, but did not use the research findings in practice (Brett, 1987; Coyle & Sokop, 1990; Pettengill et al., 1994). In these studies it was not determined if nurses who were in the stages of awareness and persuasion had access to all of the information needed to use the innovation in practice. In a research utilization study, Bostrom and Wise (1994) found that increasing accessibility to research reports through computer technology increased nurses' use of research findings, thereby enhancing the innovation diffusion process.

Innovation diffusion is the process whereby a new idea is communicated over time among members of a social system. According to Rogers (1983), this process has four distinct components: the innovation, communication channels, time, and the social system. The social system contains three subsystems: the resource system, the client system, and the change agent system. Members of the resource system possess expertise about a specific innovation. Individuals who will benefit from adopting an innovation constitute the client system and are the potential adopters of an innovation. Change agents make up the third subsystem and act as links between the members of the resource system and members of the client system, the adopters.

An individual proceeds through the five phases in the process of adopting an innovation (Rogers, 1983). During the first phase, the individual acquires knowledge about the innovation and a general understanding of how and why it works. Next, the individual weighs the benefits of the innovation to him- or herself. In the third phase, the individual decides either to use the innovation or to reject it. If a decision is made to use the innovation, the individual actually implements the innovation in the fourth phase. Finally, in the fifth phase, the individual seeks reinforcement for the innovation decision and may discontinue using the innovation if confirmation does not occur.

Knowledge Utilization and Informatics

Another important consideration in developing an innovation that increases nurses' use of research content is knowledge of *informatics*. Graves and Corcoran (1989) defined informatics as "a combination of computer science and information science designed to assist in the management and processing of nursing data, information, and knowledge to support the practice of nursing and the delivery of nursing care" (p. 3). In the science of informatics, *information* is used as a generic term that includes data, information, and knowledge (Graves & Corcoran, 1989). Information has the attributes of accuracy, timeliness, and utility (Graves & Corcoran, 1989). In the clinical setting, the utility of information to nurses depends on the nurses' perception of the quality and the relevance of the information to the patient experience. These characteristics determine the value of the information to the individual nurse. The quality of the information is determined by the effect that its use has on patient outcomes. The relevance and quality of information, therefore the utility, is obscured if the methods for accessing the information are not considered. Therefore, accessibility to research findings is proposed here as an essential component of research-based knowledge utilization by nurses in the practice setting.

This chapter describes a management innovation undertaken to diffuse the knowledge that sensory information reduces the distress experienced by patients during diagnostic procedures. Information about patients' experiences during diagnostic procedures is unavailable to nurses because of their lack of exposure to the diagnostic experience and their lack of knowledge of diagnostic tests due to the high rate of change in technology. In this project, the innovation included both the information that nurses could use in preparing patients for procedures and the use of computers to access the information in the clinical setting. The innovation was developed with three assumptions: (a) Nurses are not aware of the research on sensory information; (b) if nurses are aware of the effect of sensory information, they are not aware of specific sensations that patients experience during a specific procedure; or (c) nurses do not have access to the sensory information.

THE INNOVATION

The project, initiated at a 450-bed hospital and ambulatory clinic in an academic health center, was designed to assist nurses in using the knowledge related to the effect of concrete, objective information on patient responses during diagnostic procedures. The innovation involved using the hospital mainframe computer to provide all staff nurses with access in their clinical settings to sensory information about diagnostic tests. Two nurses developed the innovation and led the project, which involved representatives from all diagnostic departments and information management.

A survey of nurses confirmed the need for information about diagnostic procedures that could be used for patient teaching. Although the nurses surveyed identified a need for information about the diagnostic procedures, they were not aware of the research about the type of information that helped clients cope better during the diagnostic procedure.

Challenges Encountered

The innovation presented three challenges. First, the sensory information had to be collected from those who had access to the patients' experiences during the procedures. Next, the information had to be organized and transformed into a common format and then stored centrally in a computer system. Finally, the availability of the information in the computer system and retrieval process had to be communicated to the nurses.

To address the first challenge, a plan for collecting the information about patients' experiences was developed by the organization's project specialist for the nursing department and by directors of all diagnostic departments. The participating departments included radiology, clinical laboratory, radiation medicine, endoscopy, cardiac studies laboratory, and vascular laboratory.

An interview guide was developed to collect information about patients' sensory experiences during their diagnostic procedures. Individuals performing the procedures provided concrete objective descriptions about the sensations that patients verbalized during and after the procedures. The personnel in the diagnostic departments were instructed to list only those sensory experiences reported by at least half of the patients, to use descriptive terms in the patients' language rather than evaluative terms, and to identify the cause of the sensation. They were also asked to describe the procedure room and to give the time required both for the procedure and for interpretation of the results. To assist those completing the data collection tool, the project leaders included an article describing what type of preparatory information was helpful for patients and why (McHugh, Christman, & Johnson, 1982). Information was obtained on 35 different tests or procedures. An example is displayed in Table 7.1.

The second challenge was to transform the information into a common format and make it accessible to nurses in all patient care areas. First, to transform the information, the responses to the instrument were analyzed for reading comprehension level. This was done to ensure that patients could

TABLE 7.1 Example of On-Line Diagnostic Information

Name of procedure:	Arteriogram
Why it is done:	To check the blood flow in the arteries, to see if there is narrowing or if there is bleeding outside the artery, to see if the artery has a weak spot in it, and to see if the artery was malformed at birth.
How long it takes:	Varies from 1 to 3 hours.
Where the procedure occurs:	Radiology Department
What the procedure room is like:	An M.D. (Radiologist) performs the arteriogram. Registered Technologists are present. The room is well lit while you are prepared for the arteriogram. During the exam the lights are turned down—much like watching T.V. in the dark. You will lie flat on a hard table (table has small foam pad). Monitoring equipment—pads on chest for EKG, Band-Aid-type probe will be taped to one of your fingers, and you will have a blood pressure cuff on one arm. Exam equipment is moved as needed to obtain your pictures. Most films are done on a "TV Set."
What happens:	A cleansing solution that is placed on your groin is cool/cold. You will feel a needle stick when the IV is started. You will feel pressure in groin when angiography needle is first inserted. You will hear "bings," "tings," "ka-chungs," and maybe whirring sounds as the X rays are taken. You will feel a hot/warm flushing feeling as the contrast is given for the pictures. You should feel it in the area being examined; head, abdomen, or legs. You will have brief discomfort when head is positioned for taking the films due to taping a certain way to get the best pictures of the arteries in question.
Why you feel what you feel:	The cleansing solution is cool because it contains some alcohol. Needlesticks—an I.V. will be started (if not already done so), and you will experience a needlestick in the groin area as the numbing medicine is given. Pressure is felt as the artery is entered. (The needle and catheter are about the size of the lead in a wooden pencil). The warm sensation is experienced when the contrast is given, because it has to be given rapidly to catch the blood flow on film. This sensation passes quickly.
What you will feel afterward:	You may be slightly groggy if relaxing meds were given. You will feel pressure applied to your groin area for 10-15 minutes after the exam; this is to be sure the artery is not leaking. Tired of lying flat— arteriograms require you to lay flat for 6-8 hours after the exam, to protect the artery puncture site. Your vital signs will be checked frequently for the first few hours after the exam.
How long it takes to interpret test:	Results are reviewed as the test is performed. The exam is officially interpreted within 24 hours. Written report is available in 3-7 days.

understand the information in both its printed format and when used by the nurse for verbal explanations. The information was edited, formatted, entered into a word processing product, then converted to an ASCII file and transferred to the mainframe. An index listing all of the procedures was developed to facilitate the nurses' selection of information they needed for a specific patient.

The hospital mainframe computer was used as the vehicle for making the information accessible. All nurses in the inpatient and outpatient clinics have access to computer terminals located at each hospital nursing station, charting room, diagnostic department, and clinic workstation. From these terminals, nurses can use a help reference application to obtain nursing department policies and guides, hospital formulary, and department response time standards. The sensory information content and index were added to the computer's help reference menu.

Once the innovation was formulated, diffusion of the innovation presented the third challenge. Diffusion included informing the nurses about the utility of sensory information in preparing patients for tests and procedures and use of the computer to access the sensory information in their clinical settings.

DIFFUSION OF THE INNOVATION

The developers initiated the innovation diffusion process by communicating to the change agents and the client system groups as described in Rogers's social system framework. The innovation developers served as the resource system.

The developers used the formal nursing organizational structure to communicate the innovation in the inpatient nursing organization. The hospital nursing department consists of seven clinical division directors and 30 clinical nurse managers responsible for the 950 registered nurse employees. Clinical division directors were viewed as sources of support for the diffusion process, not as change agents. They received an overview of the project.

The clinical nurse managers were selected as the change agents for currently employed nurses, members of the client system group. The change agents received an explanation of both the new procedure and the relevance of its content, as well as copies of the instruction sheets and a list of all the diagnostic procedures that could be retrieved. In addition, the nurse managers/change agents were requested to explain the relevance of the sensory information and to distribute the instructions to the staff nurses on their respective units.

A different process for diffusion was developed to communicate the innovation to newly employed nurses during their orientation. All new nurses attend a 1½-hour computer training program as part of their orientation. The trainer for these classes, a member of the information management staff, was selected as the change agent for this group. The trainer was asked to add the content on accessing the sensory information to the training program.

A different organizational structure exists in the outpatient clinic component of the social system. The physician-managed outpatient clinics employ approximately 50 nurses and have no formal nursing organizational structure.

Because of the absence of a formal structure, the developers approached the clinic nurses, that is, the client system, directly. The developers explained the relevance of the information and demonstrated the retrieval process to the nurses at their computer workstations. The nurses received copies of the instructions as a reference for ongoing use of the innovation and for distribution to nurses not present for the demonstration.

EVALUATION OF THE INNOVATION

Management innovations require as systematic an evaluation as do clinical innovations (McCloskey et al., 1994). The developers evaluated the extent of use of the sensory information 1 year after the introduction of the innovation. Summative evaluation of the level of adoption, the benefits, and the costs of the innovation, gives evidence of the achievement of a successful outcome.

Level of Adoption

Rogers (1983) identified four variables that affect the level of adoption of an innovation: relative advantage, compatibility with what exists, complexity, and observability of outcomes. Because the innovation concerned diffusion of information, it was also important to include variables that influence the utility of information—quality, relevance, accuracy, accessibility, and timeliness (Graves & Corcoran, 1989). These variables combined with questions about the extent of dissemination of the innovation formed the structure for an interview guide developed for the evaluation (Table 7.2).

Twenty-eight nurses from 12 medical-surgical units and six nurses from three outpatient clinics were interviewed to determine the level of adoption of the innovation. Nurses on medical-surgical units were chosen because they routinely send patients for diagnostic tests and procedures.

The interviews revealed that the majority (79%) of the hospital nurses did not know that the sensory information was available on-line. Those who did know that the information was available were clustered on 6 of the 12 units. None of the hospital nurses who knew about the on-line sensory information and how to access it had learned about it from the clinical nurse manager, the change agent selected for the current employee group. In fact, the nurses learned of the innovation either during their new employee orientation or from another nurse who had just completed that orientation. After discovering that none of the nurses learned about the innovation from their unit managers, the developers queried the managers to determine the steps they used to communicate the innovation. All six managers employed one-time verbal or written announcements aimed at the staff as a group. Two managers gave individual

TABLE 7.2 Innovation Adoption Questionnaire

1. Are you aware that information about what a person experiences during a diagnostic procedure is available on the computer?
2. Have you ever needed or been asked by the patient/family for this information?
3. What effect do you think this information about sensory experiences has on a patient during the diagnostic procedure?
4. How did you find out about this information?
5. How did you learn to get into this information on the computer?
6. How frequently do you use the information?
7. On a scale of 1 to 5, rate the degree of complexity of getting the information.
8. Do you use the computer to access other information? What kind?
9. How did the patient or family respond to the information?
10. Is this an improvement over what you had before? Rate the amount of improvement on a scale of 1 to 5.
11. Was the information relevant?
12. Was the information easily accessible?
13. Was the information accurate?
14. Was the information timely?
15. Have you discussed this information with your colleagues?

demonstrations to a few of their staff members. None of the managers initiated any follow-up communication about the innovation.

In the outpatient clinic, the nurses recalled being shown how to access the on-line information, but none had used it since being shown. They cited two reasons for non-use: (a) lack of participation in the communication with physicians about procedures patients would undergo and (b) inability to recall how to access the information.

Those nurses who knew about the innovation were asked to provide more details about variables that affect the level of adoption. *Relative advantage* addresses the adopter's perception that the innovation is better than what previously existed. Prior to the innovation some nursing units had medical-surgical textbooks available, but nurses could not find specific sensory-related information experienced by patients during diagnostic procedures in these references. Nurses were asked to rate the relative advantage of on-line availability over what they used prior to the innovation on a scale of 1 to 10. All nurses, except the new graduates who had no prior experience, rated the innovation as a vast improvement. In addition, they found the information to be quickly obtainable and accurate.

Compatibility is the degree to which an innovation fits with the adopter's existing values, past experiences, and current needs (Rogers, 1983). To determine if nurses perceived the process as compatible with their current use of the computer, nurses were asked what other information they accessed on the computer. The process for accessing sensory information is similar to the process for retrieving nursing policies. Those who used the computer to access on-line policies also accessed the on-line sensory information, illustrating the compatibility of function with past experience. These nurses also valued the innovation as relevant to their practice.

Complexity refers to the difficulty in using an innovation. The majority reported that the process for accessing the information was easy to perform. However, if the procedure was not repeated frequently, the steps became more difficult to recall.

Observability of outcomes concerns the visibility of the consequences of the innovation (Rogers, 1983). To get an idea of observable outcomes from the innovation, nurses were asked how patients and families responded to the information. They described patients' responses as very positive, citing that patients liked the simple language, having written information, and receiving printouts for themselves and their family.

Benefits of the Innovation

The benefits of the innovation for nurses were related to the variables affecting utility of the information: *quality, relevance, accuracy, accessibility,* and *timeliness.* Nurses based their perceptions of quality, relevance, and accuracy on positive feedback from patients and families. Nurses stated that patients and families liked the information because it was plain, simple, and easy to understand. Patients particularly liked having a printed copy to refer to later and to share with family members. It was beyond the scope of the project to measure the direct benefits to patients resulting from receiving the sensory information, that is, decreased stress levels during procedures. Benefits to the patient in affecting levels of stress have been demonstrated in the past two decades of research on sensory information.

Nurses' responses about the accessibility and timeliness of the information were based on their actual experiences. Nurses stated that they could not find this type of information in medical-surgical textbooks available on their units. In fact, not all nurses had access to updated references on their units. Nurses stated that by using the computer, they could access the sensory information "in a matter of seconds."

Costs

In any innovation diffusion process, it is important to conduct a cost-benefit analysis. No equipment costs were incurred for additional hardware and software, as existing systems were judged to be adequate. The costs incurred for this project related to personnel time spent in data collection, data transformation, and uploading the information into a system for centralized access. Approximately 16 hours were spent on data collection by employees in diagnostic departments, 8 hours in data transformation, and another 16 for uploading. This translates to less than $1,500.00 in labor expenses.

Lessons Learned

The goal of the project was to provide nurses with access to research-based information. Feedback from the nurses in the client system, however, indicated that none of the diffusion efforts expended by the nurse managers/change agents resulted in adoption of the innovation. It is important to determine why diffusion efforts succeed or fail. Analysis of this diffusion process based on Rogers's model evoked three fundamental reasons for the lack of adoption.

First, in order to inform and persuade the client system, change agents must be confident in their understanding of the value of the innovation. Change agents must also be technically competent in their use of the innovation. The innovation project leaders spent little time developing these qualities of an effective change agent in the managers. In fact, one manager stated that she did not feel confident in demonstrating the use of the innovation to a staff member; consequently, the diffusion process ended. In future innovations involving computer technology, resource agents must ensure that the change agents develop a high degree of technical competence.

Rogers (1983) asserted that change agents often assume that innovations will succeed and therefore do not take responsibility for follow-up throughout the innovation adoption process. Change agent success is related to the degree of effort expended in communication activities with clients. In this diffusion process the managers made staff aware of the innovation but did not follow through to facilitate the adopters' progress though the other stages of adoption. Perhaps this resulted from the managers' lack of understanding of the innovation diffusion process. Change agents should be taught not only the innovation, but also the stages for the assimilation of an innovation. This knowledge assists the change agent in responding to the individual characteristics and needs of the client system, as well as the developmental events of the diffusion process that occur over time. They then can use informed strategies to promote the success of the adoption. Nursing leadership/management texts include an overview of the classical diffusion theory, but this may not be sufficient. Further, current managers may not have been exposed to this recent nursing management literature.

Another potentially important reason for the failure of the manager as change agent may relate to the lack of homophily between the managers and the staff nurses. *Homophily* is the extent to which individuals share common

characteristics. Rogers (1983) asserts that homophily strengthens the communication link between change agents and client systems. Managers and nursing
staff perform different functions; consequently, they attach different meanings
to an innovation. Lack of shared meaning may affect the priority that the
manager gives to disseminating the innovation.

In order to attain homophily, the change agent must be closely connected to
the clinical application of an innovation. It follows that the effective change
agent should be an identified leader within the clinical user group. The move
toward a greater business emphasis for the manager role and the transformation of clinical specialists to case managers has created a void in *clinical*
leadership roles. It is incumbent upon nursing leaders to delineate a clinical
infrastructure that will provide effective change agents within the peer group
of adopters.

In this diffusion process, those who were aware of and using the innovation
were new employees or staff taught by new employees. New employees learned
of the innovation in the computer training component of their general orientation. This finding raises a question about who should introduce new innovations to existing staff. Traditionally, the staff development department has
introduced new patient care technology innovations to existing nursing staff.
As information technology innovations become integrated into nursing process activities, it will become imperative that staff development specialists
develop competence in informatics.

SUMMARY

Research utilization requires locating a body of knowledge that can be
synthesized and its clinical meaning extracted. For nurses to use the extracted
knowledge, it must be disseminated to the point of care. Nurses' individual
attitudes, the practice environment, and access to the literature serve as barriers
to nurses' use of research findings (Barnsteiner, 1995). The computer can
address the issue of accessibility, but the critical factor will be informing nurses
of the quality of the knowledge, its relevance to their practice, and how to
retrieve it.

As the use of computer information systems to support practice grows, the
need for information specialists also increases. Efforts by the information
specialists to make new knowledge accessible to nurses in clinical practice will
be most effective when the diffusion model is integrated into the planning,
implementation, and evaluation process. The study of diffusion theory will be
essential in the preparation of nursing information specialists.

Diffusion theory also has implications for other components of the nursing organization. Particular attention must be given to the role of change agents, the essential link in the communication of an innovation. Their understanding of the innovation adoption process, as well as their involvement in each stage of development, is crucial to the success of innovation projects. Designing effective change agent roles within the nursing infrastructure will strengthen the links among innovator, technology, and nurse and thereby narrow the gap between research-based knowledge and clinical practice.

REFERENCES

Barnsteiner, J. H. (1995). *Knowledge utilization: Leadership strategies.* Paper presented at the Sigma Theta Tau, Delta Psi Chapter Research Day, Lexington, KY.

Bostrom, J., & Wise, L. (1994). Closing the gap between research and practice. *The Journal of Nursing Administration, 24,* 22-27.

Brett, J. L. (1987). Use of nursing practice research findings. *Nursing Research, 36,* 334-349.

Christman, N. J., Kirchhoff, K. T., & Oakley, M. G. (1992). Concrete objective information. In G. M. Bulechek & J. C. McCloskey (Eds.), *Nursing interventions: Essential nursing treatments.* Philadelphia: W. B. Saunders.

Coyle, L. A., & Sokop, A. G. (1990). Innovation adoption behavior among nurses. *Nursing Research, 39,* 176-180.

Graves, J. R., & Corcoran, S. M. (1989). An overview of nursing informatics. *Image: Journal of Nursing Scholarship, 21,* 227-231.

Johnson, J. E. (1974). Effects of accurate expectations and behavioral instructions on reactions during a noxious medical examination. *Journal of Personality and Social Psychology, 29,* 710-718.

McCloskey, J. C., Maas, M. L., Huber, D. G., Kasparek, A., Specht, J., Ramler, C., Watson, C., Blegen, M., Delaney, C., Ellerbe, S., Etscheidt, C., Gongaware, C., Johnson, M., Kelly, K., Mehmert, P., & Clougherty, J. (1994). Nursing management innovations: A need for systematic evaluation. *Nursing Economics, 12,* 35-44.

McHugh, N. G., Christman, N. J., & Johnson, J. E. (1982). Preparatory information: What helps and why. *American Journal of Nursing, 5,* 780-782.

Pettengill, M. M., Gillies, D. A., & Clark, C. C. (1994). Factors encouraging and discouraging the use of nursing research findings. *Image: Journal of Nursing Scholarship, 26,* 143-147.

Rogers, E. M. (1983). *Diffusion of innovations.* New York: Free Press.

CHAPTER 8

Expanding the Communication Structure in a Nursing Research Center

Eve L. Layman
Sandra G. Funk
Brenda K. Cobb

The Center for Research on Chronic Illness was established to advance knowledge about chronic illness in vulnerable people and to inform nursing practice through dissemination of the Center's research findings. Because of the limitations of traditional dissemination methods and the advantages offered by newer electronic communication mechanisms, the Center has chosen to share its research with the nursing research and practice communities through the World Wide Web on the Internet. This chapter describes the steps the Center took in developing the Web pages, the costs of doing so, strategies selected to evaluate and maintain the pages, and methods for publicizing the availability of the pages. Implications for nursing administrators are addressed. It is hoped that this example will stimulate other nursing centers and institutions to develop their own Web pages, thereby enriching the knowledge base of nursing practice, facilitating the conduct of research that is responsive to the quickly changing health care environment, and opening communication channels between and among care providers and researchers worldwide.

The Center for Research on Chronic Illness in Vulnerable People (CRCI), funded by the National Institute of Nursing Research at the National

Institutes of Health (NIH), was established at the University of North Carolina at Chapel Hill School of Nursing to foster the development, conduct, and dissemination of research on preventing and managing chronic illness. Currently, chronic illness is the major cause of mortality and morbidity in the United States (U.S. Department of Health and Human Services, 1992). More than half of the American population has one or more chronic illnesses, and for almost a third of these individuals, the ability to perform normal daily activities is limited by illness (Lambert & Lambert, 1987). Children are also affected by chronic illness: 31% are estimated to have a chronic illness or condition (Newacheck & Taylor, 1992). The research of the Center focuses on those who are most vulnerable to chronic illness: the poor; the young and the elderly; those living in rural areas without ready access to health care services; and minority groups. There is a critical need for cost-effective interventions to assist these chronically ill persons to maintain or recover function and to promote independence and enhance their quality of life; it is also critical to help others remain healthy. The Center provides support, training, and collaborative opportunities to its investigators to facilitate the conceptualization, design, and testing of interventions to prevent and manage chronic illness.

DISSEMINATING THE WORK OF THE CENTER

The overarching goals of the Center are to advance knowledge and to inform nursing practice through its research. To achieve these goals, the Center is committed to disseminating the results of its conceptual and methodological advances and its research findings to both the research and the practice communities. Both traditional and new electronic methods of dissemination are used by Center investigators to share their findings. Although the traditional methods of conferences, presentations, and refereed publications are important avenues to reach the research audience and gain the peer review necessary to evaluate scientific merit, they involve lengthy delays in the dissemination of findings—the time lag from research completion to publication is often as much as 2 years (Baker, Liberman, & Kuehnel, 1986; Funk, Tornquist, & Champagne, 1989). In the meantime, other researchers are proceeding apace, often unaware of the related research that has already been conducted. The science becomes fragmented, the use of methodological advances is delayed,

AUTHORS' NOTE: This work was supported in part by Grant #P30 NR03962 from the National Institute of Nursing Research, the National Institutes of Health.

The authors would like to thank Center Director Dr. Joanne Harrell, Ms. Janet Tysinger, and Ms. Elizabeth Tornquist for their invaluable guidance in the development of both the Web pages and this chapter.

and duplicative efforts to develop instruments and interventions are under-taken. The time lag also means that researchers do not respond as quickly as they need to in building the science to guide practice in a rapidly changing health care environment. Further, publications present studies as isolated efforts (Ament, 1994), with little dialogue or joint exploration of the meaning of findings by the research community. Conferences are more timely and provide opportunities for dialogue, but they reach relatively small audiences.

These traditional methods of research dissemination are even more prob-lematic for reaching the practice community. It has long been documented in the literature that established techniques present formidable barriers to effec-tive access to research findings. The time lag to publication is a critical problem (Bohannon & LeVeau, 1986; Funk et al., 1989). Clinicians need the results of the research now, not 2 years from now when an article is published. Further, the studies that are published are often not readily accessible to practicing nurses—accessibility is limited by distance from comprehensive health sciences libraries; the dispersion of relevant literature throughout multiple journals, books, and reports; and the time needed to search these sources and synthesize the information (Bostrom & Suter, 1993; Funk, Champagne, Wiese, & Torn-quist, 1991; Stetler, 1994). Research results are more quickly available at con-ferences, but shortages of time and travel monies make regular conference attendance impossible for most nurses in practice (Briones & Bruya, 1990; Pettengill, Gillies, & Clark, 1994). Finally, research reports often lack the specificity needed to guide implementation of research-based innovations. More effective means of sharing research with clinicians and more clinician-researcher dialogue are needed to overcome these barriers (Baker et al., 1986).

THE INTERNET AS A DISSEMINATION TOOL

Newly available electronic communication networks such as the Internet represent a dissemination method that has the potential to reach both re-searchers and clinicians quickly, extend information to those in rural areas, collect the relevant literature in one place, present both ongoing and completed research in accessible language, and facilitate researcher-to-researcher and researcher-clinician dialogue (Barron, 1995; Crosby, Finnick, Ventura, & Erdley, 1995). Specifically, using the World Wide Web, an information system that runs over the Internet, computer users connected to the Internet can "visit" Internet sites, view text and graphics information, identify and link to related sites or information, and communicate with others on the Internet. Informa-tion on the Web is presented in the form of Web pages—computer files of text, graphics, and audio and video information coded in a language called Hypertext Markup Language (HTML) that controls how the information is displayed and that provides a means to link between Web pages. The user employs a software package called a browser (e.g., Netscape) to access the Web and view Web pages (see Glossary in Table 8.1).

In the past 5 years, the Internet has experienced exponential growth— becoming increasingly available to academic institutions, health care organizations, industry, community agencies, and the public throughout the United States and internationally (Milio, 1995; Sparks, 1993). The Internet reaches both rural and urban areas and allows individuals to access a broad array of information at the network's many sites and to communicate with individuals and institutions worldwide. The Center for Preventing and Managing Chronic Illness is making use of the Web to disseminate information on its research. While the current focus of much of nursing informatics is on the development of databases for clinical and research use (Ozbolt & Graves, 1993), the primary purpose of the communication technology adopted by the Center is not storage of raw data for analytic purposes, but the distribution of the latest study results and their interpretation. While benefits of the Internet as a communication tool are still unfolding, other researchers have also used the structure to promote researcher collaboration and information dissemination (Cerf, 1995). This information management strategy requires only the adaptation of existing technologies and linking to an existing system. This chapter describes the Center's development of electronic communications over the Internet in order to stimulate other organizations to incorporate nursing informatic technologies in the dissemination and utilization of research.

DEVELOPMENT OF THE WEB PAGES

The Center decided to explore the possibility of using the Internet to overcome the disadvantages of more traditional methods of disseminating research and to meet its goals of (a) informing the nursing community of the Center's existence, (b) rapidly disseminating to researchers and clinicians the Center's latest research on chronic illness, and (c) facilitating their communication with our researchers to stimulate collaboration and use of the research in practice. The Center selected the Internet as its primary electronic communication technique because it is the largest computer network; reaches millions of users across the world; provides users with almost instantaneous access to the Center's information; and has a ready means, through electronic mail (e-mail), to communicate with the Center's investigators. The Center was equipped with the necessary computer resources to undertake this project,

Table 8.1 Glossary of Key Terms

Term	Definition
browser	a program that converts World Wide Web hypertext files to readable format, and provides a mechanism for viewing and moving between the documents stored on separate and often widely dispersed network servers.
CRS	Communication Resource Specialist: staff member responsible for information dissemination through electronic mechanisms.
HTML	Hypertext Markup Language: one type of hypertext used in World Wide Web documents in which tags are incorporated into the text of the document to create a distinct format.
hypertext	a specialized communication protocol using embedded symbols to format files, making them readable through software applications such as browsers.
Internet	a linked group of computer networks extending throughout the world that enables information to be disseminated to individuals or groups through rapid interactive processes.
network	a communication system made up of individual computers that can directly exchange information through specialized protocols; network complexity can increase by connecting networks to other networks.
URL	Uniform Resource Locator: the address by which others can locate documents or other Internet-associated communication systems.
Web pages	documents written in hypertext format that convey information through specialized computer programs; the initial page of a Web page series is designated the "home page" and functions as an index from which other linked documents can be rapidly located.
World Wide Web	an electronic linkage system that uses hypertext language to present and connect Web files stored on Internet servers.

SOURCE: Adapted from Howe, 1996, and *Internet Unleashed*, 1995.

including a high-end personal computer, an Internet connection via the University's network, and software for programming and viewing Web pages.

The development of the Web pages required policies and procedures, design and layout, content, and a time line for completion of the work. Policies and procedures were established to specify the parties responsible for preparing each aspect of the Web page content, the nature of that content, who would review it, and who would have rights and responsibilities for accessing and altering the computer files. A communication resource specialist (CRS) was hired to implement the plan.

In the design phase, expensive graphics were avoided by creating an electronic version of the Center's logo in several sizes for the introduction to the Center's home page, for the header of each subsequent page, and for trailer icons to provide a link back to the home page. A common background color, consistent with the University's color scheme, was selected for all pages, and bullets and lines of varying colors, shapes, and sizes were used to provide structure and to stimulate interest across the pages. When graphic links were needed to provide connections to other pages, text links were also provided to accommodate users with older browsing software that does not include graphics support. Page length was kept to a minimum for the main pages, so viewers could get an overall sense of the Center before delving into detailed presentations.

The most critical decisions were those related to the content of the Web pages. Content needed to include general items such as an introduction to the Center, the Center's purpose, its location, a description of the Center's activities and resources, and the way to communicate with Center personnel. Detailed descriptions of its research projects were needed to meet the Center's dissemination goals. Figure 8.1 depicts the final structure selected for the pages. The Center's first page, called the "home" page, introduces the Center's logo, welcomes the viewer to the Center, provides an overview of the Center's Web pages, and gives the Center's mailing address and e-mail address (see Figure 8.2) (the home page can be accessed at URL: http://www. unc.edu/depts/crci). Each main heading on this home page is a link to Web pages that provide additional detail about the Center. "Background Information" links to a page outlining the Center's aims, its definition of vulnerable populations, and Center operations. "The Four Cores" (Figure 8.3) describes the Center's cores and subcores, the goals of these units, and the services they provide. The section, "CRCI Scientists," lists the Center's core scientists, investigators, consultants, and advisory committee members.

The heart of the Center's pages is the presentation of research studies being conducted by its investigators, including both large-scale supporting studies, funded by NIH, and smaller pilot/feasibility studies, funded by the Center. Decisions needed to be made about the depth and breadth of information to be provided. While full text of research proposals would provide the greatest amount of detail about a study, the sheer volume of information would overwhelm the reader. Complete descriptions of intervention protocols might be desirable for the clinician, but would be premature, since studies were still evaluating the interventions' effectiveness. Therefore, the Center decided to present detailed summaries of its research studies that highlight key empirical and theoretical underpinnings of the research, study methods and measures, results to date, and the significance of the findings. To facilitate use by clinicians, summaries are written clearly, minimize jargon, and emphasize the meaning of the findings over statistical testing (Tornquist & Funk, 1993). Full references to key related works by the investigators are provided to assist readers with learning more about the research topic and the foundations of the ongoing study. Access to the investigator is available through the Center's e-mail address on the home page if questions arise. Collectively, these research presentations

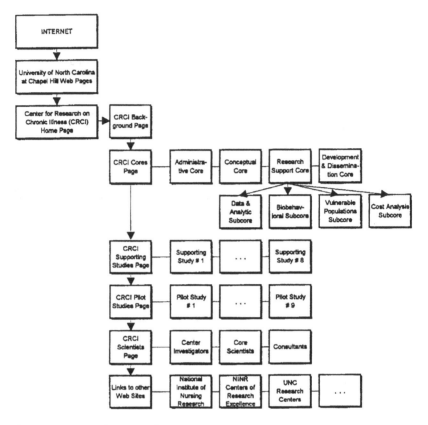

Figure 8.1. Center for Research on Chronic Illness Web Page Structure

present a more comprehensive and timely look at chronic illness than can be found elsewhere in single articles, edited books, or conference presentations.

Multiple rounds of review and editing by the Center directors, project manager, CRS, editor, and researchers were done to ensure accuracy of substance, adequacy of coverage, and clarity of presentation. As page content became ready, the CRS coded it in hypertext, creating a bank of pages that, upon completion, were uploaded to the University's UNIX machine for Internet access. The pages were then pilot tested by multiple users to provide an additional check on the HTML coding and the transfer to the University's UNIX machine. After final edits, the Center announced the availability of the Web pages to all Center personnel for review and feedback.

An initial time line of 6 months was established for creating the Web pages. Mounting an effort of this magnitude, however, required a year. The work involved more than 20 people with differing schedules; required multiple

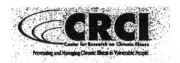

The Center for Research on Chronic Illness in Vulnerable People

Welcome to CRCI

The Center for Research on Chronic Illness in Vulnerable People (CRCI) at the School of Nursing, University of North Carolina at Chapel Hill (UNC-CH), is one of 6 research centers funded by the National Institute of Nursing Research (NINR) at the National Institutes of Health NIH(NIH) to promote excellence in nursing research. Activities of the multidisciplinary team of researchers are coordinated through the leadership of Dr. Joanne Harrell, Director of CRCI, and Dr. Sandra Funk, Associate Director of CRCI

These webpages were created to inform researchers and health care providers about the CRCI and the current state of the research it sponsors. Core activities, individual CRCI scientist's research, and CRCI announcements, are found in the following pages. Although the content contained in these pages focuses on research conducted at the University of North Carolina at Chapel Hill, we hope other readers previously unfamiliar with health care research who read through the CRCI webpages will find something useful.

More information about CRCI

- □ Background Information
- □ The Four Cores of CRCI
- □ CRCI Supporting Studies
- □ CRCI Pilot/Feasibility Studies
- □ CRCI Scientists

You may write to any of the CRCI directors and scientists in care of the Center at:

Center for Research on Chronic Illness
University of North Carolina at Chapel Hill
School of Nursing, Carrington Hall, CB#7460
Chapel Hill, NC 27599-7460

You are invited to share in CRCI's scientific activities by returning to CRCI's webpages frequently.

Select underlined text or icons to:

Continue with more CRCI information:

Core Groups Support Studies Pilot Studies CRCI Scientists

The staff and investigators of CRCI look forward to your comments. Please send email to us at: crci@unc.edu

Figure 8.2. Center for Research on Chronic Illness Home Page and Link to "The Four Cores" Web Page

rounds of review; and was affected by the vagaries of computer hardware, software, and network connections.

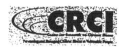

▦ The Four Cores of the CRCI

The work of the CRCI is organized into four cores:

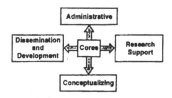

● <u>Administrative Core</u>

    Directors: Joanne Harrell, PhD, RN, and Sandra Funk, PhD

    The Administrative Core provides overall management of the CRCI,
    disseminates information about the Center, manages the pilot study grants
    program, and maintains Center resources.

● <u>Conceptualizing Core</u>

    Directors: Merle Mishel, PhD, RN, FAAN and Julie Fleury, PhD, RN

    Scientists in the Conceptualizing Core work to develop theoretical frameworks
    for studying the prevention and management of chronic illness in vulnerable
    people through critical analysis and synthesis of current knowledge.

● <u>Research Support Core</u>

    Directors: Joanne Harrell, PhD, RN, and Michael Belyea, PhD

    The Research Support Core facilitates the development and conduct of CRCI
    research through methodological, measurement, and statistical consultation
    and education.

● <u>Development and Dissemination Core</u>

    Directors: Margaret Miles, PhD, RN, FAAN, Sandra Funk, PhD, and Elizabeth
    Tornquist, MA

    The Development and Dissemination Core facilitates the development of new
    investigators, manages a research fellowship program for minority
    investigators, and aids in the dissemination and use of research findings from
    Center studies.

Select the underlined subcore titles above for specific subcore information.

Select underlined text or icons to:

Continue with more CRCI information:

<u>Core Groups</u> <u>Support Studies</u> <u>Pilot Studies</u> <u>CRCI Scientists</u>

Figure 8.3.   Center for Research on Chronic Illness "Four Cores" Web Page

PUBLICIZING THE WEB PAGES

While there are millions of Internet "surfers" who might find the Center's pages in their wanderings through the Internet, concerted efforts have been made to inform the nursing community of the availability of the Center's Web pages on the Internet. In order to reach the nursing research and practice communities that are the focus of its dissemination efforts, the Center is advertising its Web pages in handouts at nursing research and practice conferences, including the address on business cards, having the University and the School of Nursing include links to the Center in their Web pages, and requesting that Yahoo, Alta Vista, and other Internet search services include the Center in their data banks. The National Institute of Nursing Research, which funds the Center, also includes a link to the Center in its Web pages: other major nursing organizations such as Sigma Theta Tau have been asked to do the same.

MAINTAINING THE WEB PAGES

To maintain currency of the research on the Web pages, they are updated every 3 months. All Center investigators are alerted to the need to update their research summaries and publications. To minimize error and confusion, all edits are routed through the CRS, who has the primary responsibility for the Web pages. The CRS makes the coding changes to the computer files. As with initial content, updates are reviewed, edited, and approved by the Center directors, project manager, CRS, and an editor.

To assist Center investigators and document incoming communications from viewers of the Web pages, e-mail, related phone calls, and paper mail are routed through the Center. The CRS reviews the incoming mail, routes it to the directors or study investigators as appropriate, and follows up with these individuals to ensure that responses are sent in a timely manner.

COSTS OF CREATING AND MAINTAINING WEB PAGES

Creating and maintaining Web pages involves both physical and human resources. A relatively well-equipped personal computer (in 1998, a Pentium processor with 16 megabytes of memory) capable of running the latest browser program and connected to the Internet either directly or indirectly through a network is necessary. Many institutions, such as universities, provide Internet access free to their constituents; others may need to obtain services from a commercial Internet server. Software needs include an HTML editor to facilitate coding of the Web pages (versions of which can be obtained by accessing shareware on the Internet) and an Internet browsing program.

Human resources include the time of individuals with substantive knowledge to write, review, and edit the content of the pages, and the time of an individual with Web page expertise to code the page content in HTML and prepare the files for Internet access. The time required depends on the complexity of the pages being written. In addition, if professional graphics, audio, or video are desired, costs for professional development of this material may need to be included.

EVALUATION OF THE WEB PAGES

Several methods have been designed to evaluate the effectiveness of the Web pages in disseminating research results and communicating with researchers and practitioners. The most direct method for measuring the number of readers accessing the Center's Web pages is the monitoring program on the home page that counts the number of Web page "hits" and stores the Internet user ID of the person accessing the pages. The counter is monitored monthly to establish frequency patterns and to list the file of user IDs. Although this does not provide details about the individuals who view the pages, or the extent to which the remaining pages are read, the number of hits does indicate how visible the pages are to others, and the user IDs provide information about repeat users and distribution of users across Internet sites. A user survey requesting information on the perceived utility of the pages and the background of the user has been structured into the Web pages for those who wish to provide feedback to the Center. In addition, a Center e-mail address enables users to provide direct feedback about their use of and views about the Web pages. The CRS and Center investigators also log all inquiries received as a result of information disseminated through the Web pages. Materials disseminated and collaborative relationships established through contacts facilitated by the Web pages are documented and tallied.

FUTURE OF THE CENTER'S WEB PAGES

As time permits, the Center will be adding new and exciting features to its Web pages. As the final results of Center studies become available and are published in peer-reviewed journals, the Web pages will be adapted to present these more detailed findings. We will also have the opportunity to go beyond what is presented in the traditional research journal. Here, on the Web pages, the details of a successful intervention protocol can be presented along with a reprint of the full text of the research article. Researchers wishing to replicate the intervention and clinicians wishing to implement it would have access to much richer detail than any current forum provides. Further, this is the point at which dialogue with the investigator becomes critical. Clarifying the protocol, understanding acceptable adaptations, and knowing the applicability to various populations can be readily explored with the investigator through the Internet. As individuals contact Center investigators with questions about how to implement an intervention, how to adapt an intervention for their setting, or how best to administer a new assessment technique, these questions and the investigators' responses will be featured in a question-and-answer section for each study. Clinicians beginning an implementation project and researchers wishing to replicate the study can review this information to learn what problems others have encountered and what solutions the investigators suggest. The experiences and suggested solutions shared with us by others will be featured as well.

The Web pages that we describe here are, we hope, just the beginning of a comprehensive compilation of the latest research on chronic illness. As we publicize the availability of the Center's Web pages and encourage others doing work in this critical area to share their findings via the Internet, we will build links to their Web pages into the Center's Web pages. Thus, by visiting the Center's pages, the researcher or clinician will have ready access to a rich array of the latest information to guide further research or practice. As the group of participants grows, the opportunities for sharing strategies for effectively incorporating findings into practice will grow as well, moving practice forward at a much faster pace than is possible with more traditional research dissemination methods.

IMPLICATIONS FOR NURSING ADMINISTRATORS

As Center researchers begin to communicate through the Web pages the human experience of chronic illness and variations in human response to illness, particularly in vulnerable people, nurses will gain new insight into their practice regardless of its location. Nurse administrators and leaders of professional practice in various health care settings can influence the use of this new technology in establishing clinician-researcher relationships that will ultimately benefit patients (Aydollette, 1988; Stetler, 1992).

The Center's Web pages could be particularly useful to directors of nursing services, because the information contained in these pages reflects the most current understanding of how particular chronic illnesses are experienced by various populations and how that experience affects their response to nursing interventions. Innovative nursing programs modeled after those interventions tested in Center-sponsored studies can then be customized to unique settings.

Not only can the Center's Web pages aid the work of nurse administrators, but they can be useful to an organization's clinical researchers. Most of the current Center studies are testing nursing interventions in community settings. The conceptual frameworks on which these studies are based can provide clinical researchers in diverse settings a broader understanding of the factors that influence a patient's response to nursing interventions. Thus, creative solutions to special population health problems encountered in specific health care settings can be generated.

As nurses throughout an organization become familiar with Internet resources and skilled in navigating the Web pages, they may identify ways in which the communication tool may advance their own work. That is, they may decide that a Web page will enhance the professional practice of their nursing groups in a manner similar to that experienced by the Center. Results of clinical nursing studies can be quickly disseminated to a wide audience and increase the potential for establishing mutually beneficial relationships. In addition, clinical guidelines that evolve from specific studies or that have been success-fully adapted for specific settings can be shared with other organizations. Nursing groups that independently write Web pages can use the Internet not only to publicize their group's work, but also to link their pages with others, placing their efforts in a broader framework. Following the Center model for centralizing information on chronic illness and its prevention or management, other nursing groups can create extended information sources using their Web page as a focal contact.

Currently, most academic institutions provide nurse researchers access to the World Wide Web and other Internet tools at no cost to the institution. Health care centers associated with educational facilities, using a university system, can also affordably access the Internet. Through projects such as AJNetwork and the Physicians Access the Internet (Chi-Lum, Lundberg, & Silberg, 1996; Sparks, 1993), rural health care systems are being offered training and computer support services that may include Internet access. The likelihood that these financial resources will continue to provide Internet access at reduced or no cost is minimal, however. Since the largest growth in Internet membership in the past has been in commercial organizations (Ellsworth, 1995), it seems reasonable to conclude that connection to and use of the Internet will eventually require purchasing access through commercial com-munication firms. Nurse administrators will be instrumental in determining whether their institutions incorporate the Internet as a communication and information mechanism for nursing service (Aydollette, 1988; Simpson, 1996).

The decision to connect the organization with the world of electronic communication requires commitment to incorporating the various techniques into everyday practice and acquiring necessary computer equipment and software, consultants, and trainers. In addition, work time must be allocated to nurses to practice their newly acquired skills and to create new avenues for using electronic communication techniques in their unique settings (Ozbolt & Graves, 1993; Simpson, 1996).

VISIONS AND VENTURES

We can only begin to imagine the future of this technology and the advantages it will provide for information dissemination. Already, information shared via Internet includes animation, sound clips, and video presentations. Three-dimensional graphics are now possible, as is real-time communication. Journals are now available to be read on-line, and library holdings and compilations of journal articles can be searched via the Internet. New articles are being published solely on the Internet, and processes are being developed to provide peer review of these materials (Harnad, 1993). Investigators are already exploring the possibilities of conducting research directly on-line—delivering interventions, assessing subjects, and communicating the results via the Internet. As these possibilities unfold, important issues of data security, subject rights, and sound research design and methodology arise. The scientific, practice, and informatics communities will need to collaborate to address these pressing concerns and to ensure that the integrity of the science and the quality of its dissemination is maintained, and hopefully enhanced, by these new technologies.

CONCLUDING REMARKS

As described above, use of the Internet overcomes many of the barriers to traditional methods of research dissemination. Information can be shared more quickly and fully; multiple sources of information can be linked together to provide depth and breadth in a topic; dialogue between investigators and other researchers and clinicians is facilitated; and as contacts are established, collaborations become possible. It is hoped that the example we present here of the Center for Research on Chronic Illness's creation of Web pages and use of the Internet to disseminate information about the Center and its research will stimulate others in the nursing community to share their research and practice outcomes with others through the Internet. As the volume of nursing information on the Internet grows and we begin to categorize, catalogue, and evaluate it, nurses will have more ready access to the information they need to conduct cutting-edge research and practice more effectively. The science and practice of nursing are thus enhanced, and quality of care and patient outcomes are improved. The possibilities are virtually limitless.

REFERENCES

Ament, L. A. (1994). Strategies for dissemination of policy research. *Journal of Nurse-Midwifery, 39*, 329-331.

Aydollette, M. K. (1988). The nurse executive in 2000 A.D. In M. Johnson (Ed.), *Series on nursing administration* (Series on Nursing Administration, Vol. 1, pp. 2-13). Menlo Park, CA: Addison-Wesley.

Baker, T. E., Liberman, R. P., & Kuehnel, T. G. (1986). Dissemination and adoption of innovative psychosocial interventions. *Journal of Consulting and Clinical Psychology, 54*, 111-118.

Barron, B. (1995). Colleges and universities on the Internet. In *The Internet unleashed 1996* (pp. 864-888). Indianapolis, IN: Sams.net Publishing.

Bohannon, R. W., & LeVeau, B. F. (1986). Clinicians' use of research findings: A review of literature with implications for physical therapists. *Physical Therapy, 66*, 45-50.

Bostrom, J., & Suter, W. N. (1993). Research utilization: Making the link to practice. *Journal of Nursing Staff Development, 9*, 28-34.

Briones, T., & Bruya, M. A. (1990). The professional imperative: Research utilization in the search for scientifically based nursing practice. *Focus on Critical Care, 17*, 78-81.

Cerf, V. G. (1995). *Computer networking: Global infrastructure for the 21st century* [on-line World Wide Web]. Available: http://www.cs.washington.edu/homes/lazowski/cra

Chi-Lum, B. I., Lundberg, G. D., & Silberg, W. M. (1996). Physicians accessing the Internet, the PAI Project: An educational initiative. *Journal of American Medical Association, 275*, 1361-1362.

Crosby, F., Finnick, M., Ventura, M. R., & Erdley, W. S. (1995). Readiness of nurses for electronic networking for quality assessment and improvement. *Journal of Nursing Care Quality, 10*, 40-45.

Ellsworth, J. H. (1995). The idea of the Internet. In *The Internet unleashed* (pp. 4-7). Indianapolis, IN: Sams.net Publishing.

Funk, S. G., Champagne, M. T., Wiese, R. A., & Tornquist, E. M. (1991). Barriers to using research findings in practice: The clinician's perspective. *Applied Nursing Research, 4*, 90-95.

Funk, S. G., Tornquist, E. M., & Champagne, M. T. (1989). A model for improving the dissemination of nursing research. *Western Journal of Nursing Research, 11*(3), 361-367.

Harnad, S. (1993, October). *Implementing peer review on the Net: Scientific quality control in scholarly electronic journals.* Paper presented at the International Conference on Refereed Electronic Journals: Towards a Consortium for Networked Publications, Winnipeg, Manitoba.

Howe, D. (1996). *On-line dictionary of computing* [on-line World Wide Web]. Available: http://wombat.doc.ic.ac.uk/cgi-bin/foldoc?Free+On-Line+Dictionary

Internet unleashed (2nd ed.). (1995). Indianapolis, IN: Sams.net Publishing.

Lambert, V. A., & Lambert, C. E., Jr. (1987). Psychosocial impacts created by chronic illness. *Nursing Clinics of North America, 22*, 527-533.

Milio, N. (1995). Beyond informatics: An electronic community infrastructure for public health. *Journal of Public Health Management Practice, 1*, 84-94.

Newacheck, P. W., & Taylor, W. R. (1992). Childhood chronic illness: Prevalence, severity, and impact. *American Journal of Public Health, 82*, 364-371.

Ozbolt, J. G., & Graves, J. R. (1993). Clinical nursing informatics: Developing tools for knowledge workers. *Advances in Clinical Nursing Research, 28*, 407-425.

Pettengill, M. M., Gillies, D. A., & Clark, C. C. (1994). Factors encouraging and discouraging the use of nursing research findings. *Image: Journal of Nursing Scholarship, 26,* 143-147.

Simpson, R. L. (1996). Technology: Nursing the system. Managing the social and behavioral impact of technology change. *Nursing Management, 27*(6), 26-49.

Sparks, S. M. (1993). Electronic networking for nurses. *Image: Journal of Nursing Scholarship, 25*(3), 245-248.

Stetler, C. B. (1992). Nursing research and quality care. In M. Johnson (Ed.), *Delivery of quality health care* (Series on Nursing Administration, Vol. 3, pp. 191-207). Boston: C. V. Mosby.

Stetler, C. B. (1994). Refinement of the Stetler/Marram model for application of research findings to practice. *Nursing Outlook, 42,* 15-25.

Tornquist, E. M., & Funk, S. G. (1993). How to report research with clarity, coherence and grace. *Journal of Emergency Nursing, 19,* 498-502.

U.S. Department of Health and Human Services. (1992). *Healthy people 2000, National health promotion and disease prevention objectives: Summary report.* Boston: Jones and Bartlett.

PART III

Tips From the
Information Innovators:
Creating Change Across
Health Care Settings

This section is devoted to case studies that describe innovative use of technology across different populations in a variety of health care settings.

In the first chapter of this section, Behrenbeck, Timm, Gudlin, and Briske describe the implementation phase of a clinical information system at a large internationally renowned Midwestern tertiary care center. The description of this comprehensive point-of-care implementation project includes project management, computer system preparation and installation, staff education, actual implementation steps, and project evaluation. This case study is particularly noteworthy because it focuses on point-of-care technology and highlights critical success factors and lessons learned during such a project.

In Chapter 10, Brokel, Hawkos, Getman, Schumacher, and Schwichtenberg describe a case study that highlights a challenge calling for unique solutions for coordinating care in integrated delivery networks (IDNs). This case study is particularly remarkable because it addresses the clinical and nursing information system needs within a rural, sparsely populated region. The chapter clarifies actual information system needs in an IDN, implications for system interfaces, use of common language and implications for system design, and the management of network information systems in an IDN.

In Chapter 11, Owens-Vance, Kraft, and Lang focus on the development and implementation of the nursing information components of a fully integrated, patient-focused clinical information system that is the basis for the Veteran's Health Administration (VHA) electronic patient record. These authors briefly describe the VHA information system structure, the administrative and clinical aspects of the nursing information management system, and user training. Also included are postimplementation evaluation data and plans for future developments.

In Chapter 12, McGuire describes a case study that focuses on providing support to patients and caregivers in their home environment using computer technology. This chapter offers a brief description of the use of ComputerLink to reduce caregiver social isolation and increase decision-making confidence for providing in-home care for patients with Alzheimer's disease. A detailed description of a cost-effectiveness evaluation of this innovation is a strength of this chapter.

Kowalski extends one's understanding of the relevancy of minimum data sets to the management of nursing home facilities and corporations in Chapter 13. She summarizes several case studies using the Minimum Data Set (MDS) mandated through the Health Care Finance Administration (HCFA). Corporate evaluation of data, quality indicator development and evaluation, and additional management uses of the MDS are highlighted. Moreover, Kowalski includes process and system considerations, cost information, and case mix reimbursement and classification impacts of the MDS. Clearly, the MDS has moved the long-term industry ahead; it is now the industry's responsibility to use the data to advance nursing care.

In the final chapter, the tremendous capability of information systems to impact care delivery in community settings is highlighted by Bargstadt. He highlights the function of information systems in capturing data from three perspectives: individual clients, groups of clients, and the community as client. He concludes the chapter by addressing data and information issues for meeting both the financial and clinical needs arising from service to individuals, groups, and communities.

CHAPTER 9

Organizing Project Implementation for Success: A Major Medical Center Case Study

Julia G. Behrenbeck
Jane A. Timm
Doreen J. Gudlin
Susan A. Briske

This case study focuses on the implementation phase of a clinical information system on two medical/surgical nursing units at a large Midwest tertiary care center. The implementation included bedside workstations in every patient room and other locations throughout the units. Because of the point-of-care access, printouts of the patient care record were completed only upon transfer to a noncomputerized unit or discharge.

A multidisciplinary steering and user group provided structure for the project. Project managers from the Department of Nursing and Information Services provided accountability for implementation. The project managers facilitated communication with the software vendor to develop work plans and address issues. Benefits evaluation included structured patient interviews, user questionnaires, collection of quality indicator data, identification of system performance measures, and collection of system use data. Resource support for education and go-live coverage was also evaluated.

The data definition was defined through review of institutional practice and national standards. Nursing classification systems were studied and included in the system configuration.

BACKGROUND

The long-range goal of this project was to improve patient information management for direct care providers in the hospital setting. The initial focus was on patient information collected by nurses. Efforts to meet this goal began in 1988 when a Nursing Informatics Committee was convened. A nursing system model was developed as part of a feasibility study (Behrenbeck et al., 1990). The model provided an overview of information management for the Department of Nursing by identifying data classes created or used in nursing. These were organized according to the processes that act on the data during work activities.

In a parallel effort, the manual documentation system was studied to improve and streamline the system. A new, more efficient manual documentation system was implemented in the summer of 1994. This system uses a structure for documentation of professional nursing practice that includes the North American Nursing Diagnosis Association (NANDA; 1994) taxonomy and the Nursing Interventions Classification (NIC; McCloskey & Bulechek, 1996).

Building on both the system analysis and the manual documentation study, the functional requirements for an electronic system were outlined. A Request for Proposal (RFP) was sent to approximately 40 computer vendors. Seven vendors were selected to demonstrate their system using a structured format. Based on the user and technical evaluation, three systems were chosen for more in-depth evaluation.

A proposal to pilot one of the three systems was submitted for approval. During this process, it was clear that broad institutional involvement was lacking, cost-benefit questions were outstanding, and fit with the institutional goals for development of an Electronic Medical Record (EMR) was questioned. Thus, an institutionwide task force was formed with nursing, physician, and administrative input. In early 1993, the group recommended moving ahead with a pilot study of a point-of-care system.

An interdisciplinary group worked for 1 year to prepare the chosen computer system for implementation. In the meantime, the organization made a decision to partner with another vendor for the development of an institutionwide Electronic Medical Record (EMR). Based on this decision, the computer system available through the second vendor was evaluated for implementation in the hospital setting. After a thorough, structured evaluation, a unanimous decision was made to conclude the pilot study with the first vendor. Although

AUTHORS' NOTE: We would like to acknowledge the enthusiasm and commitment of the nursing staff on the two implementation units; and the teamwork and leadership of the various groups and committees that contributed to this project.

there were advantages and disadvantages with each vendor product, consistency with the development of the EMR was the deciding factor. A proposal was approved for implementation with the new vendor on two medical/surgical units.

PROJECT OVERVIEW

The system was implemented in the spring of 1995 on a 24-bed orthopedic surgery unit and a 23-bed medical unit. Both units have a combination of private and semiprivate rooms. One bedside workstation was mounted on an articulating arm in each room to support the point-of-care concept that was key to this project. Manual nursing documentation was converted to an electronic point-of-care system. Unit secretaries maintain census information and transcribe physician orders into the system. Nurses document patient vital signs, assessments, problems, interventions, and outcomes using the system. The data entered into the system are available for the multidisciplinary health care team to review on-line at workstations located in the patient room or throughout the patient care unit. The patient record is printed upon transfer of the patient off the unit or at discharge.

The project focused on a quick implementation that would maximize ability to provide input to the next release of the software. Interfaces to other hospital systems were therefore not developed for this implementation. However, because documentation of medication administration constitutes a considerable piece of the patient record, a window to the pharmacy system for on-line documentation of medication administration was implemented on one of the units.

Successful implementation was dependent on the following steps, which were carefully planned and orchestrated:

- Project management
- Computer system preparation
- Hardware and software installation
- Go-live preparation
- Education
- Implementation
- Project evaluation

Our experience with each of these steps will be detailed in the remainder of this chapter.

PROJECT MANAGEMENT

This project was managed jointly by three project managers. From nursing, one person focused on the vendor product implementation while the other focused on the enhancement of an in-house pharmacy system for the on-line documentation of medication administration. The Information Services (IS) project manager focused on the entire implementation from a technical perspective. User and technical cross-departmental project teams were organized into three groups. A Steering Group, chaired by a physician, provided project direction; a Clinical Work Group defined the configuration and operational flow with the new system; and a Technical Team worked closely with members of the engineering, networking, facilities, and vendor teams to carry out the implementation. An executive group made up of the chairs and secretaries from these three groups met periodically to direct and coordinate activities among the groups. Time lines were developed and reviewed frequently.

SYSTEM PREPARATION

The data definition was defined through review of institutional multidisciplinary practice and national standards. Nursing classification systems were studied for inclusion in the system configuration. Our goal was to utilize existing standardized language systems throughout the documentation process; to reflect linkages among problem statements, interventions, and outcomes; and to provide input to further development of the classifications.

Our initial design included components of NANDA and NIC in the on-line care plan application. This application linked NANDA and NIC but was not integrated with the flowsheet application. Because the care plan application did not support the Nursing-sensitive Outcome Classification (NOC; Maas, Johnson, & Moorhead, 1996) format, this approach was revised when we became a test site for NOC. The care plan application was replaced by an on-line care plan flowsheet that incorporated NANDA and NOC (see Figure 9.1). Nursing interventions, which currently are not in a standard language format, are documented on a second on-line flowsheet (Figure 9.2). A third on-line flowsheet was developed for the documentation of patient/family education.

The new care plan flowsheet was divided into standard categories. Within each category, there was a subsection for nursing diagnosis, NOC outcomes, and an ongoing assessment. Nurses added appropriate nursing diagnoses and outcome rows to the flowsheet for each patient. Advantages of the new design included: greater flexibility in the charting terms, increased integration of care planning with other documentation, and a more acceptable user interface.

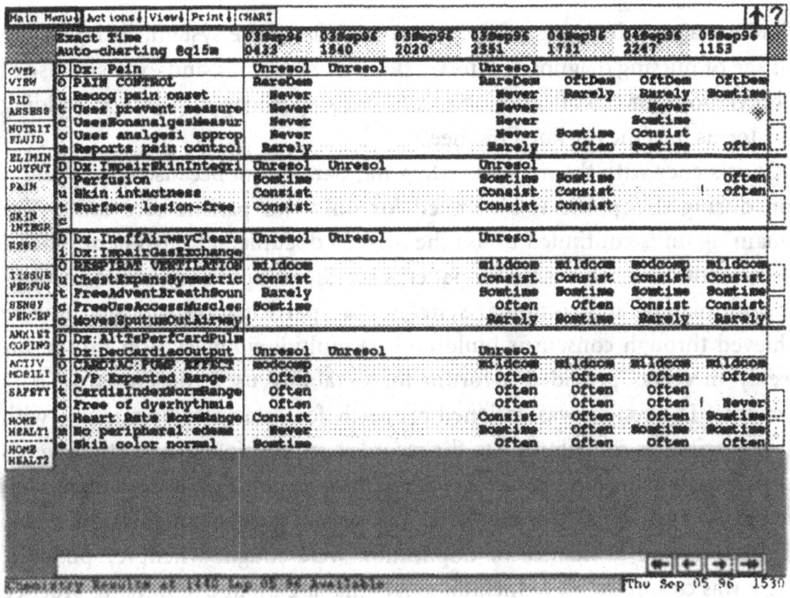

Figure 9.1. Care Plan Flowsheet

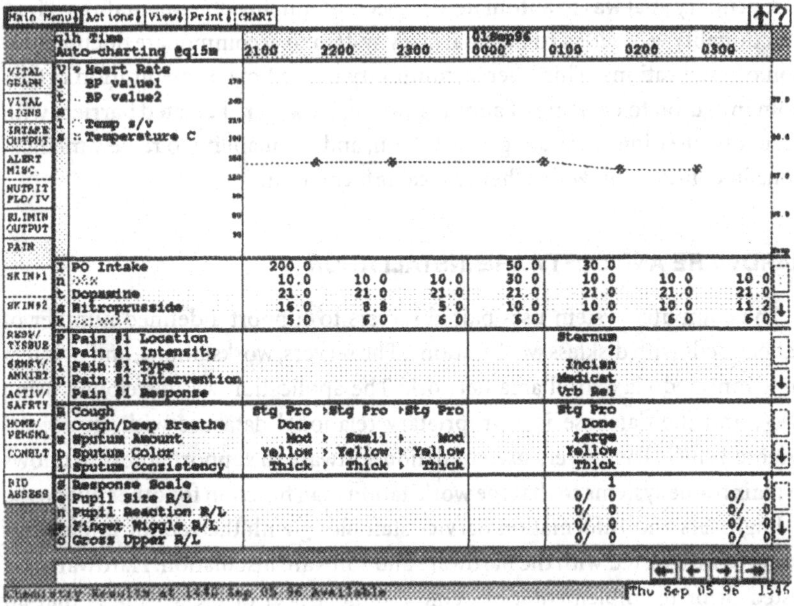

Figure 9.2. Medical/Surgical Flowsheet

Disadvantages, which are related to limitations of the system, included: no linkage of nursing diagnoses, interventions, or outcomes, and excessive use of abbreviations for classification terms. A next step is mapping and/or building NIC terms into the on-line flowsheets.

Consistency with the manual system was paramount because implementation during this phase was planned for only two patient care units. The remaining units continued to use the manual documentation system. Therefore, practitioners who cared for patients across multiple areas would encounter both manual and computer systems. User participation and buy-in were achieved through consensus building in a multidisciplinary user group. Biweekly meetings provided a forum for obtaining user consensus on data elements. The system was designed primarily for data entry by nursing, with other disciplines contributing to the record as appropriate to meet their needs but primarily using it for review of patient information. Respiratory therapists, dietitians, and social workers used the system for documentation. Standardization and avoidance of duplication were sought whenever possible. There was commitment to including data that are unique to nursing practice while identifying similarities and supporting data needs of other disciplines. For example, common terminology and abbreviations were used for assessments and treatments that were similar for respiratory therapists and nurses.

A primary goal was to automate all aspects of nursing documentation. Thus, functionality was added to the pharmacy system to accommodate documentation of medications. This offered continuity in the flow of medication orders from initiation to charting of administration. However, it created barriers with a separate user interface, a separate log-on, and the inability to review medications in conjunction with other clinical information.

HARDWARE AND SOFTWARE INSTALLATION

The computer system uses paired servers to support a defined number of patient beds with diskless workstations. The servers, workstations, and printers are connected via a local area network. The application was developed using C++, and the database is a proprietary relational database with an object-oriented shell. The servers use emulation software to support access windows to mainframe systems so that the workstations can function for other purposes.

Engineers and Information Service staff along with the vendor implementation team assisted with the hardware and software installation. Hardware was tested prior to implementation. One unique aspect of the setting is that an engineering team is responsible for providing ongoing support for the hardware in conjunction with the vendor. Spare parts are kept on site so that engineering staff can replace some system components during failures without having to wait for the vendor.

Providing bedside access presented several challenges. A team of representatives from the Nursing, Engineering, Systems and Procedures, Ergonomics, Facilities, and Information Services departments was formed to define the bedside system requirements. Care provider, patient, visitor, space, and security requirements were identified. Space in patient rooms and flexibility in moving the system were major considerations in defining the following requirements: The nurse must be able to sit or stand while using the system. The system must not create a safety hazard. The system must be quiet, and the monitor light must not be bothersome at night. The arm must fold up and be out of the way when carts are brought into the room for patient transport. The equipment must be secured to prevent damage or loss.

Initially, engineers developed an articulating arm prototype for a notebook workstation. This concept was then shared with a vendor for further development. Through discussions of hardware options with the software vendor, the bedside system was defined as having an 11-inch flat panel monitor, a spacesaver keyboard with a membrane, and an ergonomic trackball. The vendor developed a double articulating arm that can move up and down as well as fold away. The arm has 18.5 inches of vertical movement and extends 42 inches from the wall. It can be customized for whatever monitor and keyboard a user decides to purchase. The arm uses a pneumatic cylinder that can be adjusted to counterbalance the weight of the monitor, keyboard, and trackball, making it easy for the user to adjust the height and position quickly. A wrist rest and handle were added to the arm for ease of use. The central processing unit (CPU) box was mounted on the head wall above the arm. This resulted in using extension cables and developing a 12-foot video cable (see Figure 9.3).

GO-LIVE PREPARATION

Utilization of a team approach was important to successful implementation. This strategy was used throughout the planning phase. Separate go-live dates, 2 weeks apart, were selected for each unit, allowing lessons to be shared during implementation on the second unit. This provided enough time for the first unit to become acclimated so resource staff could focus on the go-live of the second unit.

Procedures were developed to support the changes in philosophy, work flow, and documentation by representatives with expertise in nursing practice, education, and systems. With the coexistence of manual and computerized patient care records, the procedures were developed with reference to the

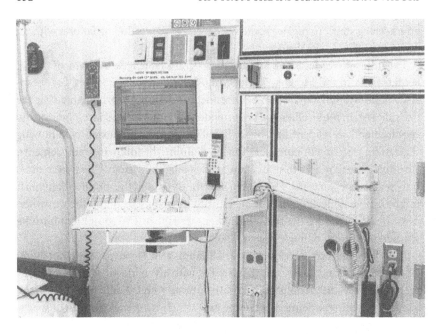

Figure 9.3. Bedside Workstation Setup With Articulating Arm

manual process and were consistent with institutional policies. They captured differences between the manual system and the computer system in areas of work flow and process, as well as details and nuances of the system. For example, procedures were written for security maintenance, downtime, care planning, and documentation of medications. The procedures were used in the education process and were made available on the two computerized patient care units.

Procedures were developed for printing of the patient record upon transfer or discharge, and as back up in case of system failure. Physicians and allied health staff review the patient record on-line during the patient's stay on the computerized unit. Printed copies of the record are not distributed to the patient's chart until discharge or transfer off the unit. Approval was obtained from the appropriate organizational groups for the format and procedures related to printed reports.

Emphasis was placed on changing work habits and organizational flow with implementation of point-of-care technology. The strength of this concept is increased efficiency in updating the patient's record and improved access to timely patient information during the care process.

The system configuration tools supported on-going testing of data definition and format as the system was being configured. Testing of the software and hardware continued during the preparation phase with assistance of the vendor's implementation specialists. A mock go-live was conducted on each unit. During this test, documentation was completed using both electronic and manual charting for one patient on each unit for 24 hours. This test provided insight into use of the bedside device, work flow, and other processes (e.g., tracking intake and output, printing the patient record, etc.). Changes in design and content were made throughout the testing, training, practice, and initial go-live.

Support from nursing management played a vital role in the success of the project. Early in the preparation phase, the necessary adjustments in unit staffing were estimated. Through a central staffing and scheduling office, staffing adjustments were made to provide adequate unit coverage during scheduled classes and practice time. It was determined that additional staff nurses would be assigned to the units for the first month after go-live to ensure integrity of patient care and to function as unit resource staff. Planning included representatives from the staffing/scheduling office and the float staff management. Nurses and secretaries were identified to be educated from float staff and other patient care units with similar patient populations. Maintaining staff computer competency and ensuring availability of computer-trained staff proved to be a challenge with implementation on only two patient care units.

Resource materials were created and strategically located on the unit for easy reference. A manual included procedures, resource staff contact numbers, and a section to log issues. Pocket-size laminated cue cards were distributed for quick reference on application navigation and use. Laminated instruction algorithms were created to streamline a cumbersome printing function for unit secretaries. System user manuals were also available on the units. Computer labels were placed on all computer workstations to distinguish them from other computers located on the units.

A support staff network was established to ensure prompt resolution of emergent software and hardware issues. The first-line support included designated unit staff resources who also participated as trainers for the classes. On-call pagers were used for contacting one of five designated nursing system experts for clinical questions and one of three information system staff for technical questions. Issues were logged by on-call staff and directed to the project managers for any necessary follow-up. Unit staff utilized the issues log to record questions and comments. Issues were reviewed at user group meetings, resolutions were proposed, and/or any necessary education identified.

Communication was important to inform groups affected by the change. It was acknowledged that patients and their families may have misperceptions and concerns about computers in the patient rooms and access to their medical information in multiple locations. A standard letter was generated that explained the point-of-care concept and management of patient information. Copies of the letter were distributed to patients and their families at the time of admission to these units. This was accompanied by an explanation from the unit staff. Communication was also provided for other departments and disciplines. This occurred through an article in the staff newsletter, verbal explanation to physicians as they made unit rounds, and dissemination of the information through the usual organizational network for such announcements.

EDUCATION

The challenge and success of any project is integration of the system through the education process. Attitudes, fears, and expectations of the system were all things that needed to be addressed. An initial time line was set giving each of the two nursing units 4 weeks for education. Approximately 170 nurses and 70 ancillary staff were trained. A preassessment survey was sent to staff to evaluate previous exposure to computers; level of comfort; preference for day, evening, or weekend classes; and willingness to work above their designated full-time equivalent (FTE). A 100% return rate on the surveys proved the investment of the nursing staff involved in the project. Computer literacy ranged from no exposure to those who were "surfing the Internet." Because we intended to utilize a train-the-trainer model for this project, it was important to design training classes for all levels of competence.

The trainers were educated on the system over a 3-day period by the implementation specialist from the vendor. The trainers included Nursing Information Specialists, Nursing Education Specialists, Clinical Nurse Specialists, management for the nursing units, and designated staff nurses from each unit. Curriculum for the subsequent training periods was designed based on the training course as well as input from the clinical work group, which had invested a significant number of hours over the previous 1½ years, tailoring the computer system to the needs of the institution as well as to the specific nursing units. Each staff RN received 16 hours of classroom instruction.

Reinforcement of the education was done through two methods: practice or mock patient charting and double charting on actual patients. Practice charting was possible through the test development system on the computer. Staff could admit a mock patient and explore the various parts of the patient chart by inputting data, changing data, discharging or transferring the patient, and readmitting. Double charting on actual patients was also set up in a couple of the patient care rooms to provide staff the opportunity to "test" the system with actual patient data. One or two 8-hour shifts were provided to each staff nurse to have the opportunity to care for one patient and trial the computer system. The manual chart was maintained and data were duplicated on the computer chart. This provided an excellent means of evaluation for the nurse and a forum to ask questions and address issues not faced in the classroom setting with scenarios.

Shortly after go-live, each staff nurse was also required to have a competency check by one of the trainers. This competency check was to be returned to the Nurse Manager to be placed in the employee's file. The competency check was a return demonstration involving all aspects of the various flowsheets of the patient chart.

Evaluation of education was assessed following the first month of use on the computer system in the unit. This amount of time was important for true reflection of the usefulness of the education process. It gave the user a chance to evaluate which aspects of education were most useful and what may have been missed or done differently. The written evaluation assessed both the classroom instruction and the practice charting, as well as the resources available to the unit during go-live. A 25% return rate was achieved on the evaluation process. Relatively little feedback was given for areas of improvement. Most were complimentary of the process and felt they were adequately prepared for a successful go-live experience.

Ongoing education needs have included two facets: (a) new staff orientation, and (b) additional float pool nursing staff to meet the needs of the units during high peak census times. An in-depth guide was constructed to assist individual preceptors on the units with the orientation of new staff to the computer system, while more formal classroom instruction was provided for the float staff for education of larger groups and for practice with scenarios. The largest problem incurred for ongoing training was the lack of training facilities. Additional computer projects under way competed for available training facilities.

A security guideline was developed to provide a systematic and consistent method of handling patient information both in the computerized paper document and the on-line record. The guideline addressed access to the computer system as well as issues of confidentiality.

A six-character password was assigned to each user and is used to access the computer system. The social security number for each user is the internal unique identifier. The system has the capability to assign read-only or read/write access, allowing differing levels of authorization. A security procedure was written to detail the process for obtaining a password to access the system. This included routine activation for new staff nurses and ancillary staff, routine activation for new physicians, activation for immediate access, record modification due to an employee name change, and inactivation for staff who either transfer off of a unit using the computer or who were to terminate from the medical center. Assignment and communication of passwords for user activation was cumbersome and resource intensive. A common log-on function is being explored for improvement of this process in future projects and implementation.

Printed reports containing patient information remain with the patient chart. Reports printed for purposes other than the permanent record are recycled after use. All recycled material is shredded prior to leaving the medical center grounds.

All security and confidentiality procedures were discussed in full with staff during the classroom portion of their education. The medical center medical record access policy was reviewed and the enforcement of disciplinary action with noncompliance was discussed.

IMPLEMENTATION

As the implementation approached, staff readiness and excitement increased. Several unit staff assumed roles as ambassadors for this change process and rallied support throughout the group. The support extended across sites with a handmade poster-size card of support from the first unit to the second unit.

Conversion to the electronic system occurred at the onset of the day shift on implementation day. On the evening prior to implementation, designated nursing and secretarial staff entered the patients into the computer system, with the assistance of the vendor implementation specialist. Patient data such as demographics, orders, care plans, and messages were transcribed into the system from the manual documents. Support staff were accessible and offered assistance to care providers during conversion to the electronic system. The planned staffing adjustments were made to support the transition. User feedback was directed to the project managers, and revisions were made to the system in a timely fashion. User feedback of a nonemergent nature was logged, reviewed by the user group, and subsequent changes made as appropriate. A newsletter was created to provide a communication vehicle for all staff. Concurrent audits of patient records were conducted and feedback was provided to appropriate staff. Retrospective audits provided information on the printing procedure, its thoroughness, and accuracy.

PROJECT EVALUATION

Many efficiencies have been realized as a result of this implementation. Unit secretaries no longer maintain manual forms for the nursing staff on the hospital chart. Handwritten physician orders are transcribed to the electronic system without waiting for availability of the single manual Plan of Care. On the surgical unit where the pharmacy system window was implemented, unit secretaries do not need to collate the printed profiles from pharmacy. Patient information is readily available to the unit secretaries through their desktop workstations.

Nursing staff are able to review and enter patient data at the point of care. This helps alleviate delays and interruptions in documentation. Documentation of patient care is more accurate in the presence of the patient because the nurse is able to record data based on real-time observations and patient interaction, compared to delayed recollection. Data are more complete and reliable because of system prompts and standardization. Patient information is readily available at multiple locations rather than by searching for the single manual hospital chart. Point-of-care access promotes increased nursing staff presence and interaction with the patient and his or her family. Patient outcomes are positively affected through automated tools for care management and caregiver communication; however, many of these gains require further development of the software and more widespread implementation of the system. Supervisory, administrative, and hospital chart review functions are better facilitated with the electronic system. Nurse managers and others have improved access and new printing capabilities. Full-time equivalent (FTE) savings related to hospital chart review functions will become achievable when the system is fully implemented in the inpatient setting. Nurse staffing will be simplified when the system is fully implemented. Current staffing on the electronic medical/surgical units is complicated by the requirement that the nurses floating to the unit must be trained to use the computer system.

Physicians and allied health professionals have not reported as many operational efficiencies related to using the system. Their documentation remains manual and results retrieval is dependent on a separate workstation. The system described in this chapter and the results system at our hospital have different front-end workstations; a future goal is to merge all EMR-related systems to a common front end. Their interaction with the system is limited to patients on the two implementation units, which requires adjusting to a new routine for reviewing the hospital chart for patients on these units. This may slow down their work flow, and some physicians have reported that reviewing patient information requires too many key strokes. The surgical unit that implemented the window to the pharmacy system for documentation of medication administration resorted to printing of this report for physician and allied health professional review. Windowing to the disparate system with separate log-on proved to be too cumbersome. Nursing staff adjusted well to the pharmacy system window and prefer it over manual documentation; however, substantial additional education and support was required. Thus, after careful deliberation, the decision was made to pursue software development with the point-of-care vendor for the documentation of medication administration on the same system.

It is anticipated that physicians and allied health professionals will realize more benefits from the system when it is available on a multipurpose workstation and integrated with the imminent EMR. Improved care management and physician order applications will also provide added value. Operational efficiencies for this group will be more achievable when the system is fully implemented in the inpatient setting. This will improve continuity of the patient record as the patient moves through the various services.

Patients reported that the bedside computer system contributes to their care and that their caregivers spend more time in their presence as a result of the system. Results of Department of Nursing quality monitoring show consistency and in some cases an increase in compliance with quality standards.

SUMMARY

The critical success factors and lessons learned during the project are summarized below:

- A strong focus on practice time and education prior to implementation, along with overstaffing during the conversion, resulted in a smooth transition to the electronic documentation system for the nursing staff.
- Project management orchestrated by nurse specialists and Information Services was key to the timely implementation and completion of project objectives.
- Team development and commitment across departments was important.
- Securing physician involvement for communication and leadership among colleagues was important.
- Physician involvement in system development and education was challenging but critical.
- Documentation of medication administration needs to be an integrated part of the system.

- Adequate training room space and facilities were important prior to and after implementation.
- Financial tracking of project cost and FTE utilization were best facilitated when the vendor, project management, and accounting agreed on a common scheme.
- Staffing of the computerized units was complicated by the fact that nursing staff floating to either unit had to be trained.
- User password administration was cumbersome and resource intensive.

Installation on these two units was the first step in preparing for expansion of the system to other hospital units. Because this application is only one part of a larger EMR effort, the front end will need to evolve to multipurpose workstations. Scalability of the software and hardware to support a large hospital setting must be resolved. An archive and data management plan for the patient information must also be developed.

REFERENCES

Behrenbeck, J. G., Davitt, P., Ironside, P., Mangan, D. B., O'Shaughnessy, D., & Steele, S. (1990). Strategic planning for a nursing information system (NIS) in the hospital setting: Development of a nursing system model. *Computers in Nursing, 8*(6), 236-242.

Maas, M. L., Johnson, M., & Moorhead, S. (1996). Classifying nursing-sensitive patient outcomes. *Image: Journal of Nursing Scholarship, 28*(4), 295-301.

McCloskey, J. C., & Bulechek, G. M. (Eds.). (1996). *Nursing interventions classification (NIC)* (2nd ed.). St. Louis, MO: C. V. Mosby.

North American Nursing Diagnosis Association (NANDA). (1994). *Nursing diagnosis: Definition and classification 1995-1996.* Philadelphia: Author.

CHAPTER 10

Clinical and Nursing Information System Needs in a Rural Integrated Delivery Network

Jane M. Brokel
Hal Hawkos
Sylvia Getman
Larry P. Schumacher
Tamara Schwichtenberg

Rural health care providers are evolving into integrated delivery networks (IDNs) in order to respond to new concepts of how best to provide health care services to our communities. Information system needs become abundantly clear as network stakeholders move rapidly forward in functional, clinical, and health care provider integration. This chapter describes one case study to identify the information needs of a network composed of 10 primary care hospitals, a secondary referral hospital, a 30-site primary care physician network, a home health agency, a senior services agency, a regional laboratory, regional rehabilitation and diagnostic technology services, regional nursing case management services, an emergency services network, and a variety of other services across 50 sites. Further, implications for system design, system interfaces, and identification and use of a common language are discussed.

Rural health care providers are evolving into integrated delivery networks (IDNs) in order to respond to new concepts of how best to provide health care services to our communities. There are increasing pressures not only to care for people when they are sick, but to improve peoples' functioning, maintain their health, and keep them well. These challenges call for unique solutions in how to integrate care to ensure that people receive the most appropriate level of quality care in the most cost-effective setting.

To accomplish this coordination of care, hospitals, physicians, nurses, and other providers have evolved from loose affiliations based upon business relationships and economies of scale to close-knit continuums maximizing economies of intellect and sharing in the risks associated with care. Some of these affiliations are asset-owned networks, whereas others are virtually integrated via contracts and other operating agreements. This evolution is happening against a backdrop of constantly shifting social and governmental changes and increasing competitive and economic pressures. Our rural geography and sparse population create an increased demand to create a truly integrated "seamless continuum of care" to meet the needs of our population base.

As a result, our network consists of 10 primary care hospitals, a secondary referral hospital, a primary care physician network with 30 sites, a home health agency, a senior services agency, a regional laboratory, regional rehabilitation and diagnostic technology services, regional nursing case management services, an emergency services network, and a variety of other health care services. The network has affiliates located in 19 counties and provides care at more than 50 sites.

Information system needs became abundantly clear as network stakeholders moved rapidly forward in functional, clinical, and physician integration efforts aimed at improving access, improving clinical quality, and reducing or controlling health care costs. Functional efforts include service and facility locations and operations, planning, human resources, education, and information management. Information systems development, being both clinical and functional, is led by a strategy team in the network of clinical leaders (three nurses and three physicians) and six functional leaders (CFO, CIO, two regional network executives, a hospital department manager, and a clinic administrator). The strategy team works from a platform plan developed in collaboration with all the stakeholders of the network with the assistance of a consulting firm.

The very nature of this diverse network, which constantly changes, places great explosive growth in our need for integrated information systems. These systems need to be able not only to transmit medical records and administrative information across geographically dispersed facilities, but also clinical practice guidelines and protocols, best practice data, medical and nursing interventions, and outcomes to improve clinical decision making and quality of care.

WHAT IS THE NEED FOR INFORMATION?

The basic premise of an integrated information system in an IDN is that the information system transcends care settings, so there is minimal redundancy in collection of data that lead to information and clinical decisions. Information on care provided in each specific setting is important to the overall management of patient care across the continuum. Today's market of information systems mirrors the current paper-based documentation systems in that the systems are typically designed to meet the needs and regulatory requirements of a specific care setting. Software vendors have targeted their products to fulfill specific needs or niches. Examples of setting-specific software include home care systems, critical care systems, cardiac cath lab systems, and systems for long-term care. These systems are designed to meet the data collection and, in some cases, decision support needs of nurses and other clinicians in these settings but fall short of meeting the needs of nursing as the patient is cared for across settings. Vital information obtained within each setting rarely is effectively communicated to other providers on the continuum. The volume of data collected at each site is overwhelming and often not formatted in a useful way for providers at other levels of care. Because of this quandary, it is often considered easier to start collecting data over again. When the client moves across all the settings in an IDN, it is easy to see the redundancy and rework this creates for nurses and other clinicians. One can argue that it diminishes quality as each new clinician or nurse who encounters the client creates interventions without the advantage of valuable assessments, interventions, and outcomes from colleagues. This ineffective use of resources contributes to redundancy and rework that results in unnecessary clinical costs and utilization, diminished value, frustration, and dissatisfaction among nurses and other clinicians.

The decision to organize a framework for the IDN begins with building relationships with the stakeholders that provide health care services. Stakeholders in the IDN incorporate perspectives of all clinicians and settings in each of the local communities. Individual representatives of the stakeholder entities collaborate to identify and prioritize the needs and common processes with the IDN. This process takes significant time because there is shared responsibility at a business and enterprise level. Networkwide meetings of nurses from acute care, skilled and long-term care, home care, clinics, and community-based services offer a means to outline Health Data Network (HDN) common processes. Meetings with therapists, business personnel, and physicians describe and define the common processes to manage patient demographics, to manage clinical results, to bill for services, and to manage a provider list. Each common process identified to outline information flow is made up of subprocesses. The management of clinical results consists of ordering clinical tests, gathering the specimen or obtaining an image, assessing the patient, analyzing the data results, and determining the treatment plan. Pathways and protocols are also common methods of designing care by multiple stakeholders and clinical professionals supported by computerized formats.

Services not provided within an IDN may require referral to tertiary centers or other care providers. Consideration must be given to the need for clinical and demographic data for these referral centers as an information system is developed.

SYSTEM INTERFACES

Today's health care information systems (IS) environment is composed of many disparate systems that were selected and implemented for specialty purposes, such as radiology, laboratory, pharmacy, and nursing. Over time, the information systems vendors with the best product in terms of system functionality have typically won out over vendors that offer a full product line but with limited functionality. Those vendors who do offer a wide application base are often very strong in the application from which the company was originated (i.e., laboratory or physician billing/AR) but have less functionality in the newly developed applications. It has become increasingly difficult for these vendors to compete on the basis of application functionality with vendors who specialize in certain applications such as pharmacy or laboratory. To alleviate this problem, many of today's top IS vendors are forming partnerships with these specialty vendors to increase product line coverage and improve system functionality. However, this "best of breed" approach has created "islands of information" that do not easily or readily interact with other systems. Interfaces have been typically developed in a point-to-point method that is both time-consuming and expensive (Figure 10.1). Each interface with another system is developed specifically for that system and has to be redeveloped for additional systems. For example, the interface between an admitting system and a laboratory system would typically send admission/discharge/transfer (ADT) information to the lab system. When a radiology or pharmacy system is interfaced to that same admission system, the interface needs to be redeveloped. This requires

144

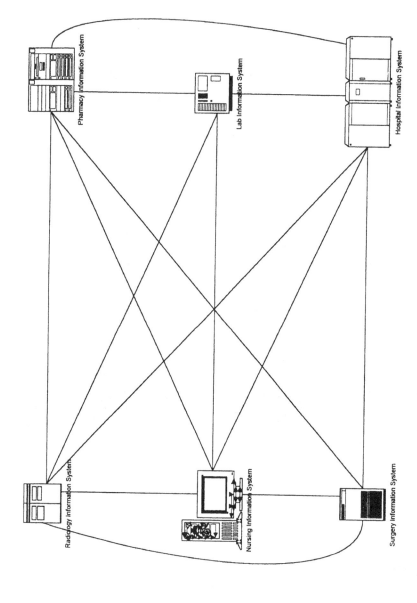

Figure 10.1. Traditional Point-to-Point Connectivity

time and money for development, testing, and implementation over and over again. Once the interfaces are developed, the ongoing maintenance of these programs is very labor intensive and expensive. Every time one of the ancillary systems changes because of a new release of the application software, these interfaces need to be modified, tested, and reimplemented for each point at which the interface is used. For example, if the admitting system is changed, the interface to each of the ancillary systems will need to be changed as well.

Interface engine technology enables health care systems to interface diverse information systems from multiple vendors. This technology eliminates the need for point-to-point interfaces between each system. The engine, which is generally a system such as an IBM RS/6000 or HP 9000, acts as a traffic cop to route and distribute information to all the systems that need it (Figure 10.2). It receives data from a variety of sources and intelligently reformats and routes the data between applications. The system uses a data mapping strategy that translates and routes information from one system to another. For example, ADT information coming from the admitting system would be sent to the engine and automatically routed to lab, radiology, nursing, and pharmacy with one transaction. Therefore, if the source system changes, the interface modifications occur only at the interface engine rather than at each of the destination systems. The engine also has the capability of reformatting transactions to meet different health care standards such as HL7, ASTM, IEEE, DICOM, or EDI-FACT. This framework enables vendor systems without health care interface standards to be interfaced to other systems.

Health care systems and provider networks are requiring better system integration. To support the continuum of care, information systems must be able to communicate information effectively and efficiently among systems and across a wide geographic area. A networked infrastructure will result in seamless access to patient information along the continuum of care. Regionalization of information systems provides an infrastructure for this communication. Information systems that used to be single-entity focused now need to be multifacility and multientity. Systems such as patient scheduling, admitting, medical records, and critical pathways will eventually become regional systems that can be accessed and utilized anywhere in the IDN through wide area networks. For example, a patient may enter into the health care system in a primary care physician office, be referred to a specialist, be admitted to the hospital, and then back to the family practice physician while being cared for at home by a home health nurse. Administrative, financial, and clinical information needs to be available to each provider along the way. If all entities are using common systems across the region, integration of those systems becomes easier and less expensive. Scheduling that patient for consultations and proce-

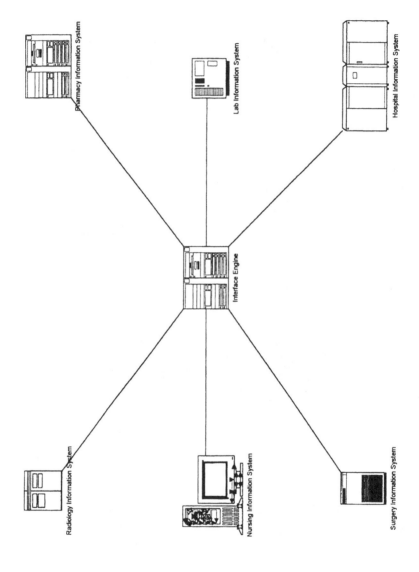

Figure 10.2. Interface Engine Connectivity

dures can be done at the point of entry into the network with immediate confirmation, rather than needing several phone calls and conversations with both the patient and the provider. The benefit of the interface engine becomes even greater at this regional level. More providers, more diverse systems and more data make the integration of systems more complex. Interface engines break down the barriers among departments, institutions, and care settings.

COMMON LANGUAGE

Common information system codes and languages that have been endorsed by international and national health care organizations provide the common communication link for stakeholders in the IDN. Decision support software applications rely on common definitions to describe diagnoses, interventions and procedures, and diagnostic tests. The logic to support decisions is dependent on the accuracy and validity of the language and definitions in use. International classification of diseases (ICD-9) and Health Care Financing Administration Common Procedure Coding System (HCPCS or CPT codes) provide a common medical language to define diseases and disorders and the interventions and tests for diagnosis and treatment. The universal use of diagnosis codes and procedure codes provides a common language to share health care information. Medical outcomes measures lack uniformity, sophistication, and wide use. Several severity-based systems exist to measure outcomes using other mortality, resource intensity indices or disease stage ratings with inpatient hospital settings. Many of these types of measurements assess only mortality outcomes and costs. Stakeholders may have to evaluate further and find applications with the potential of measuring medical outcomes across settings. Tools like the SF-36 Health Status Survey and BASIS-32 do provide the measuring of the patient's perception of outcome status over time despite care in multiple settings.

Nursing as a discipline has an evolving common language in the Nursing Minimum Data Set (NMDS) and Nursing Management Minimum Data Set (NMMDS). The NMDS critical data elements include nursing diagnoses (NANDA), nursing interventions classification (NIC), and nursing-sensitive outcome classification (NOC). A standardized assessment process that transcends all the settings is essential to the formulation of appropriate nursing diagnoses. Nursing diagnoses are then linked to NIC that defines care procedures and actions within the dimension of nursing. NOC is the first comprehensive standardized language to measure outcomes sensitive to nursing functions. The potential to link nursing-sensitive outcomes (NOC) with nursing interventions via computerized tracking affords patient progress measurements across settings in the IDN.

NMMDS is an essential set of measures that is needed across the entire IDN wherever nursing is practiced. It provides nursing executives with the information to assess what variables have affected clinical nursing outcomes. In an environment of constant change in clinical practice, managed care plan changes, and measured clinical outcomes, it is an essential data set to manage clinical care effectively in an IDN.

APPLICATION OF COMMON LANGUAGE IN THE IDN

One method for using the NIC was the development of automated clinical pathways to describe the day-to-day procedures provided in the care of inpatients, outpatients, and home care patients. The nursing intervention language—along with the CPT codes of diagnostic tests and procedures, H codes and Q codes for rehabilitation services—provides the framework for designing clinical pathways in multiple settings throughout the IDN. This provides a single plan of care for the patient as the patient crosses multiple care sites in the IDN. Nursing information systems designed to support services in all settings and with the flexibility to track patient care plans and progress in achieving outcomes toward health or maintaining health tie the nursing process across care settings within the IDN.

PathPlan 2000 is an example of a decision support software program used for flexible clinical pathway management in a variety of settings. Pathways for care in acute care and skilled care established a means to construct and outline common language procedures for tests, education, therapies, assessments, planning, and activities for populations of patients. The basic common intervention language can be refined to provide the flexible information necessary for the specific setting though categorized under common, nationally defined procedures or interventions of care. PathPlan 2000 also affords the opportunity to design life plans for populations of patients, such as well-baby pathways; health screening and education pathways for children, adolescents, adults, and the elderly; or disease management pathways for people with chronic diseases.

The transmission and access to shared plans, pathways, and protocols across a local area network and wide area network would facilitate use of common language and processes in multiple network settings. The measuring of outcomes is the responsibility of all stakeholders, because interventions in the network could be analyzed as failures or benefits to the outcome.

The challenges in creating pathways using a common language are similar to those of any policy deployment and dissemination. In using consistent and common language, the number of individuals available and knowledgeable about the process of designing and developing care pathways using computer methods and common terminology usually is limited. Knowledge of medical, nursing, and therapy diagnoses; interventions and outcomes combined with knowledge of information systems; and the utility of the system provide the sense of how best to design the use of the software program to meet the ultimate customers' needs and the immediate customers' needs. The ultimate need would be the ability to design a plan of care for the patient to achieve outcomes efficiently in the continuum of the IDN. The immediate need would be the ability to design a method understandable to the clinician for implementing and adapting the intervention plan for the patient's individual needs.

SYSTEM DESIGN

Other wide area network applications pose similar benefits for using common definitions but many challenges to meeting the patient and health care providers' needs. An integrated health care and nursing information system must be supported by a technology infrastructure and software application that traverse settings wherever and whenever care is provided to best facilitate the management of information. Wide area network HL7 standard language supports linkage and offers hope and opportunity for the united transmission of clinical data in a mobilized health care management environment. Mobile computing is no longer a luxury but a necessity, because more care is provided in a variety of locations to manage care in the community and home. On-line point-of-care documentation is essential for complete and accurate charting of care. Access to information about the patient and about the plan of care must be readily accessible and available. Real-time access to clinical reference information is necessary for planning and for evaluating outcomes.

Knowledge-based systems about medications, diseases, and so on, supported by practitioner reminders and alerts, facilitate the day-to-day decisions in nursing practice. Logical formats carry data forward to appropriate settings to support the nursing process in multiple settings. Software design that allows selecting check boxes or choosing from selection lists in drop-down menus speeds up data entry.

Two major challenges in handling nursing and health care information will be capturing discrete data that do not fit into defined categories, and common language options and data entry modes. Collection of data may include a keyboard, "pentapping" on the screen with keyboard view, handwriting, voice recognition, or combinations of these. Data collection modes will have to be easy, user-friendly, and time efficient.

Design formats will be important in settings that have data-reporting requirements, such as in long-term care minimum data set and home care requirements. Data collection on patients consists of a core set of items that are commonly used by all nurses. Data specific to settings, problems, population, and regulatory requirements are factors that affect the type and amount of other data collected from and about patients. System designs need to be flexible enough to allow users to determine their preference of screen displays to accommodate work flow in a variety of settings. Data must be able to transcend settings and be available in formats that are logical and understandable to other settings.

This specificity of practice and information needs has perpetuated the niche-specific software design. To support evaluation of nursing information, a system must be capable of displaying data in multiple views. An example of this is the ability to display the numeric values of patient temperature or to display the trends in a line graph format. Graphing capabilities provide rapid interpretation and conclusion, which is important in areas of practice that manage large volumes of repetitive data, such as critical care, and areas that manage longitudinal data, such as home care and clinics. This is important because time as an evaluation variable will be different in each setting. The home care nurse may be looking for longer-term clinical or physiologic trends than the nurse working in a critical care unit.

Nursing is a common thread in all settings within the IDN. The need for transitioning the common information through the continuum is integral in the nursing profession to provide the efficiencies and effectiveness in multiple levels of care.

SYSTEM LINKS

Links with ADT systems allow for accurate collection of demographic and benefits source information. This link to a nursing information system avoids duplicate collection of information and optimizes efficient and effective clinical and financial processes measuring utilization of resources.

Links with order entry/result review facilitate the assimilation of data for management of patient care. Nurses need to review test results such as laboratory and radiology in order to evaluate the results in the context of the presenting problems and the effect the results may have on the plan of care.

Additional links can promote efficient patient care operations, such as the billing system. A direct pass of nursing orders and interventions from documentation into the billing system should capture the charge of a care encounter. For example, based on an order for wound care, the documentation should include the supplies used and the time for nursing care associated with the dressing change and patient teaching required. The charges associated with this care would be a direct pass to the billing system and the care would be charged for. Inherent in the effectiveness of this process is standardized intervention of nursing. Only with a standardized language can the definitions of interventions be supported by the billing system. It is imperative that terms are used consistently across settings in order to determine costs of care effectively and to evaluate effectiveness of care.

Capable links with the pharmacy system allow documentation of medication administration and access to alerts for drug/drug, drug/food, or drug/allergy interactions. Information that needs to be transferred is allergies, current medications, and medication history. Patient education knowledge-based access promotes prompt education activities within a time-limited managed care environment.

MANAGEMENT

Means and methods to manage the IDN are supported by network information systems organized for wide area network applicability. A network system that allows for the ability to create procedure lists for nurses and support staff facilitates organized delivery of care. The planned interventions identified for the patient assessments and diagnosis help determine patient acuity. Based on the patient care needs/demands, the system automatically calculates acuity totals to determine staffing needs. All of this is done in the background by the system and is based on collected data; it does not require a separate, stand-alone process. This allows for appropriate skill mix ratios and provides better resource allocation. This method allows costs for direct and indirect patient care to be calculated based on the acuity and activity of nursing care.

Another management function useful in an IDN is a scheduling module that supports staffing along with the function of variance reporting among scheduled, worked, and indirect (education, meetings, etc.) hours and allows for decision-supported summary reports. The staffing function has the flexibility to accommodate various shift hours and combinations, and regular and float/registry staff. As with other interface needs, the staffing module would interface with the payroll system.

A nurse executive's legitimate understanding of what means and methods are necessary to obtain the best approach and to predict the outcomes of services across the network agencies offers hope to create a seamless continuum. A nursing information system that provides this decision support allows for trended data storage to manage services and facilitate clinical operations, marketing, and payer knowledge for decision making.

Data that have been utilized in day-to-day care must provide some utility for clinical studies and performance analysis to improve care processes and for administrative decision making regarding resources and strategic planning.

A process to manage the identification and adoption of glossaries of data definitions for the IDN and to provide uniformity in data utilized within the IDN clarifies the ongoing guidelines to standardize language in the IDN and for comparative analysis in national databases. Policy guidelines set the stage to identify data needs and data definition, select standardized national language, plan collection, and evaluate the utility of data.

The application of a common language in the IDN is the use of NIC by community-based nurse case managers. Through a home-grown software product, nurse case managers track client interventions, outcomes, and cost per member per month in a chronic illness group practice model. Eventually this documentation system will be linked to the acute care setting and primary care clinic system through interfaces that will improve communication and coordination of care efforts.

The informatics nurse specialist will be an integral coordinator and evaluator of health care information systems today and in the future. Informatics nurse specialists offer dedicated time to organizing and analyzing the functionality of information systems for clinical services. Nursing's role provides a holistic view of services over the continuum and, therefore, informatics nurse specialists can guide technical design, implementation, and evaluation of wide area network applications. Without dedication to hardware needs, software needs, and liveware needs, systems will be barriers and burdens to care. The efficiency and effectiveness of clinical care services require constant attention to build the system to manage access, collection, and use of patient information, aggregate information, and knowledge-based information systems. The informatics nurse specialist guides nursing staff, administration, and technicians in implementing systems to improve the nursing process of planning, diagnosing, intervening, and evaluating results rather than mirroring a paper-based system.

CONCLUSION

In conclusion, the benefits of a well-designed health care information system will allow the home care nurse visiting the 4-year-old child with asthma to review allergies, drug reactions, current medications and doses, latest results from previous tests, and benefits with health insurance plan using the Health

Information Network. The nurse goes to another file to identify the child's encounters with clinics and emergency centers. The nurse sees the patient was in three different cities for care and notices visits to the physician's office five times in the past 3 months. The nurse finds out that the child is just beginning preschool with 25 other students. The first 2 months of school have increased the child's exposure to colds and flu. The nurse enters the following subjective health history information and verifies and reviews the child's current immunization status: "Risks were identified with the following nursing diagnosis recommended: Risk for infection and interventions suggested for home care services. The mother expresses that she understands the two medications the child has been on but questions the benefits of the medication prescribed last night." The nurse accesses the pharmacy knowledge-based information on the new medication and helps the mother understand the common benefits and side effects. The nurse provides the mother and child with guidelines to reduce risk for exposure to colds, flu, and seasonal stressors. The nurse e-mails a message to the primary care physician on the child's latest bout with asthma exacerbation and current potential concerns with the most recent illness.

The physician's recommended intervention last night included a disease management plan for childhood asthma. Following an electronic message to the primary care physician, the physician recommends initiating a disease management plan for childhood asthma. The home care nurse receives messages and schedules a visit to the patient/family to provide further education on infection protection and follow-up assessments for asthma management. In a follow-up visit, the nurse sends electronic and voice messages to the physician and pharmacist, who have concerns about the theophylline levels with new nausea and vomiting symptoms. The nurse selects interventions and marks current status in achieving outcomes in the nursing applications. The information on the visit is collected and noted by the pharmacists and physicians.

The physician contacts the mother to have a theophylline level drawn. The test results are electronically sent to the physician, who leaves a message for the nurse to educate the mother on changes in medication suggested by the pharmacist, who monitors the trends and abnormal test results. The adjustment in medication, the flu shots, and the infection protection education are carried out by the nurse. The little child returns to school and the mother/child are asked to follow the plan for asthma disease management.

Later financial and encounter statistics can be measured to determine the administrative resource management impact. The health information network facilitates the appropriate collection, transmission, access, and use of data to health care providers. The efficiencies allow health maintenance, disease prevention, and care intervention to be taken at a variety of health care service locations in the IDN.

BIBLIOGRAPHY

Blervitt, D. K., & Jones, K. R. (1996). Using elements of the Nursing Minimum Data Set for determining outcomes. *Journal of Nursing Administration, 26*(6), 48-56.

Greengold, N., & Weingarten, S. R. (1996). Developing evidence-based practice guidelines and pathways: The experience at the local hospital level. *Journal of Quality Improvement, 22*(6), 391-402.

Maas, M., Johnson, M., & Kraus, V. (1996). Nursing sensitive patient outcomes classification. In K. Kelly (Ed.), *Outcomes of effective management practices* (Series on Nursing Administration, Vol. 8, pp. 20-35). Thousand Oaks, CA: Sage.

McCloskey, J., & Bulechek, G. (1995). Validation and coding of the NIC taxonomy structure. Iowa Intervention Project. *IMAGE: Journal of Nursing Scholarship, 27*(1), 43-49.

McCloskey, J., & Bulechek, G. (Eds.). (1996). *Iowa Intervention Project. Nursing interventions classification (NIC)* (2nd ed.). St. Louis, MO: Mosby-Year Book.

Parker, C. D., & Gassert, C. (1996). JCAHO's management of information standards: The role of the informatics nurse specialist. *Journal of Nursing Administration, 26*(6), 13-15.

Shortell, S. M., Gillies, R. R., Anderson, D. A., Erickson, K. M., & Mitchell, J. B. (1996). *Remaking health care in America: Building organized delivery systems.* San Francisco: Jossey-Bass.

♦

CHAPTER 11

Nursing Software Development and Implementation: An Integral Aspect of the Veterans Health Administration Information System Infrastructure

Bobbie Owens-Vance
Margaret Ross Kraft
Barbara J. Lang

A description of the Department of Veterans Affairs' (DVA) comprehensive hospital information system that is integrated across clinical and administrative services is provided. Attention is directed to the vital role assumed by Veterans Administration (VA) nurses in defining the infrastructure for the Veterans Health Administration (VHA) computerized information system and the design of computerized systems that address aspects of care for which nursing is accountable. Content focuses on nursing software and the implementation of computer technology for clinical and administrative decision making. Training is discussed in relation to system capacity and the responsiveness of end users to adopting computerized systems in their practice. Finally, attention is directed to the challenges involved in the implementation of a nursing information system in a multifacility health care network, including cost of system hardware as a barrier to diffusion and adoption. The chapter concludes with future initiatives that will be vital to the successful implementation of a totally computerized medical record.

In the current era of government downsizing, a rapidly changing environment of health care, and the demand for a health care focus on customer service, the Veterans Health Administration (VHA) has been involved in a major nationwide reorganization. The VHA is a network of 173 medical centers, 375 outpatient clinics, 136 nursing home care units, and 39 domiciliaries within 22 regional Veteran's Integrated Service Networks (VISNs; Department of Veterans Affairs, 1995). The VISNs are the regional health care planning networks of the VHA and provide a total continuum of health care. Information systems have become critical elements of this VHA infrastructure. Computerized information systems have been described as the "bricks and mortar" needed to bind together this complex array of services, health care facilities, and networks.

The VHA has an internally developed comprehensive integrated health care information system initially titled the Decentralized Hospital Computer Program (DHCP) and now known as the Veterans Health Information Systems Technology Architecture (VISTA). VISTA is the automated environment in VA health care facilities that supports the day-to-day operations and includes "Windows"-style and locally developed applications, as well as national VA software. The system is complemented by linkages with a number of commercially developed software programs. DHCP was originally created in a modular development process that produced a backbone of programming utilities that supported an integrated database and provided various programmer and user software tools while supporting the development process of service-specific applications. These modular software components have evolved as VISTA, a fully integrated patient-focused clinical information system that is the basis for the VHA electronic patient record. The transformation to an information system of integrated service networks provides a mechanism for improved communication and collection of data. The system will support delivery and management of clinical services for the broad customer base of more than 2.6 million patients per year (Department of Veterans Affairs, Veterans Health Administration, 1995).

The VHA employs more than 39,000 nurses, the largest group of professional registered nurses in any single health care organization. VHA nurses provide care to veterans in a variety of settings: clinics; sub-acute, acute, and long-term care hospitals; and the home. In addition to medicine, surgery, and intensive care, VHA nurses work in specialty practice areas of psychiatry, chemical dependency, spinal cord injury, rehabilitation, and geriatrics. Software development to support nursing practice had to be applicable across this entire continuum of care.

Notably, an information system for nurse users should embody administrative, educational, clinical, and quality improvement aspects of a nursing service. In addition, for the greatest benefit to patient care, hospital information systems should be integrated across services for access and use by clinicians from all disciplines. The VHA nursing software has been programmed to interface with other clinical and management packages that make up the comprehensive VISTA system.

VHA INFORMATION SYSTEM STRUCTURE

Since the commitment was made in 1982 to develop an electronic health care architecture, the VHA VISTA system has progressed from a dumb terminal/roll-and-scroll system to a sophisticated "Windows"-style system that incorporates local area networks (LANs), wireless systems, workstations, teleradiology, telepathology, and electronic patient data exchange.

The most important component of the VISTA system is its software, a set of computer programs evolving from the initial priority of discipline-specific and functional area packages into an integrated medical center system (see Figure 11.1). The Massachusetts General Hospital general-purpose programming language, developed to support an electronic hospital database management system, was selected as the primary programming language of VISTA. The Massachusetts Utility Multi-Programming System (MUMPS) is an American National Standards Institute (ANSI) standard language that was renamed "M" in the early 1990s to keep in step with later-generation programming languages. M is widely used in Europe and some Asian countries to support nonmedical applications for libraries, banking, inventory control, and scheduling systems (Lewkowicz, 1989). Through the implementation of M routines and extensive employment of a database management utility referred to as VA Fileman, DHCP has evolved into VISTA, the clinical hospital information system. The software, readily available on a CD-ROM, has been acquired and implemented in health care institutions in other countries such as Nigeria, India, England, Italy, Egypt, Finland, and Pakistan. Major use is occurring in large hospital facilities in Finland and Pakistan.[1]

The basic criteria followed in the development of VISTA software mandated that application software had to be standardized and exportable to all VA medical centers. Technical integration had to be achieved through the use of a common database, programming standards and conventions, and data administration functions. Functional integration had to be achieved through such utilities as order entry/results reporting (OE/RR) and flexible health care

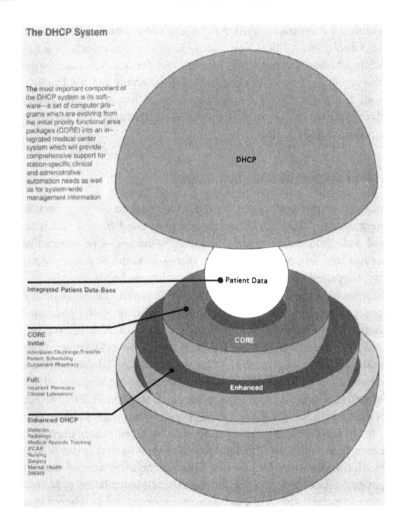

The DHCP System

The most important component of the DHCP system is its software—a set of computer programs which are evolving from the initial priority functional area packages (CORE) into an integrated medical center system which will provide comprehensive support for station-specific clinical and administrative automation needs as well as for system-wide management information

DHCP

Patient Data

Integrated Patient Data Base

CORE
Initial:
Admission/Discharge/Transfer
Patient Scheduling
Outpatient Pharmacy

Full:
Inpatient Pharmacy
Clinical Laboratory

CORE

Enhanced

Enhanced DHCP
Dietetics
Radiology
Medical Records Tracking
IFCAP
Nursing
Surgery
Mental Health
DMMS

Figure 11.1. The Decentralized Hospital Computer Program (DHCP) System
SOURCE: Department of Veteran Affairs, Veterans Health Administration (1995).

summaries. Standard data elements, timely access to data, avoidance of dependence on a specific vendor, and user-friendliness were considered necessary, and system integrity was required to protect against loss, unauthorized access to data, or both. Redundancy and duplication of data entry was avoided. The Department of Veterans Affairs is implementing a progressively intuitive, user-friendly clinical support system that consists of a totally computerized electronic patient record, a telecommunication network for complete interchange of data within each facility and network of facilities while supporting open communication to external systems. This initiative is critical to enhanced effectiveness in clinical decision making and improved patient outcomes.

The success of the VHA system was recognized in 1995 when the Computer-based Patient Record Institute (CPRI) singled out the capabilities of VISTA in support of the computerized patient record. Nursing has been, and continues to be, an integral aspect of this development process.

NURSING INFORMATION MANAGEMENT SYSTEM

The VHA nursing system addresses both administrative and clinical aspects of nursing, staff education documentation, and quality improvement data collection. The nursing software package within VISTA is designed to support planning and documentation of nursing care provided and to support nursing administration in making sound, timely decisions in the management of human and material resources for enhanced patient care services. This nursing system is made up of specific clinical and administrative modules to facilitate nursing practice across all functional areas.

Developmental History. The uniqueness of the VHA health care information system resides in its use of grassroots groups made up of administrative and clinical end users to define the software specifications for programmers to use in creating the software. Advanced practice nurses with clinical specialties, administrative expertise, or both, assumed major responsibility for writing specifications of all of the internally developed nursing software. These nurses formed a Special Interest User's Group (SIUG) that assumed responsibility and accountability for the VHA nursing software development. Specifications for the initial and enhanced versions of software releases were provided and prioritized by the SIUG with the assistance of staff at the Alpha/Beta test sites and of nursing colleagues who use the nursing software on a daily basis. The advantage of this approach included the capability to address specific nursing standards and to tailor outputs to meet specific nursing requirements while maintaining a high level of nurse user-friendliness. As discipline-specific software development moved to an interdisciplinary approach, the original SIUG evolved into an Expert Panel (EP) (see Figure 11.2). The Nursing EP with interdisciplinary membership representing such disciplines as Pharmacy, Social Work, Medicine, and Rehabilitation has continued to demonstrate leadership in defining specifications for software that will be used by clinicians. Although it is often noted that nurses and nursing practice data are frequently missing elements in hospital information systems (Ball, 1994), this was not the

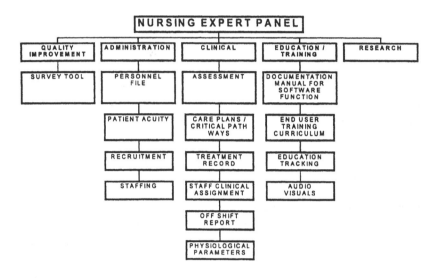

Figure 11.2. Expert Panel

case in the development of the VHA system. The Nursing System is an integral aspect of VISTA.

NURSING ADMINISTRATION MODULES

The computer may be described as a tool that enhances the decision-making capability of the nurse executive, nursing management, and clinical nursing staff. Software programs have been designed to assist in decision making and the diagnosis of management problems and to facilitate the efficient use of resources. The modules originally developed for VHA Nursing Administration include Patient Classification, Man-Hour Data, Workload Statistics, and a Personnel Database. It is possible to transfer management resource data from the mainframe through Fileman and other software utilities into personal computer (PC) spreadsheets for analysis and presentation of aggregated data. Data can then be displayed in a variety of formats, including charts and graphs that are easy to review.

Patient Classification. The first nursing software in DHCP to receive nationwide implementation was the Patient Classification module. Patients are classified daily according to their level of dependency and need for nursing care. The computerization of the patient classification system used across the VHA has facilitated real-time access to information on patient acuity, census, and related staffing requirements. Managers have the tools to review assignment patterns and make decisions about resource utilization that have greater relevance to the existing workload. Staff nurses do the patient classification, have access to the classification information, and appreciate the ease of reviewing this objective data descriptive of patient care requirements. Review of classification data over time is particularly useful in the determination of acuity/census trends used to facilitate budget projections of the number and type of personnel needed to provide patient care.

Man-Hour Data and Workload Statistics. Actual on-duty staffing by level of staff is recorded in the Man-Hour module. Direct and indirect care hours may be documented on a shift-by-shift basis. Indirect care hours can be identified as staff time spent in administration, education, and orientation activities. This module links to patient classification data and facilitates the generation of workload statistics and productivity reports. Clinical nurse managers have direct access to this information and have demonstrated a much greater understanding of the relationship between resource utilization and productivity scores. Budgeted and actual as well as recommended staffing requirements for a nursing unit, section, or service are automatically calculated and resulting variances displayed. Reports can be produced for a single shift, a day, week, month, quarter, or year. Many sites have chosen to input unit scheduled hours on a prospective basis so a projected view of unit staffing is available to supervisory staff who make decisions regarding resource reassignment. This software module has also proved to be a useful tool for retrieving staffing data for JCAHO (Joint Commission on Accreditation of HealthCare Organizations) review during survey visits.

Personnel. On-line access to the comprehensive Personnel Database provides administrators and managers with demographic and professional information about the personnel assigned to the service. Timely access to this data has improved management ability to make decisions about personnel assignments and resource utilization. The personnel profile includes such elements as demographics, educational preparation, work experience, professional license (state and renewal date), military status, certification, and dates for annual performance evaluation. Employee phone numbers are readily accessible in emergency situations. Information can be retrieved for individual or aggregate data. The VISTA nursing personnel database contains an interface that supports a link between this database and commercial staff schedulers. Many VA medical centers have chosen to automate their staff scheduling process.

A position control file monitors past, current, and future occupancy of nursing positions and documents future vacancies and reasons for vacancies. When a registered nurse's assignment is changed, the professional experience file in the staff record is automatically updated. Supervisors have access to information about probationary periods and the performance evaluation requirements for subordinates. Reminders can be generated identifying evaluation date, change in employment status, and eligibility for promotion. This system supports timely completion of evaluations and an effective personnel incentive award program.

VISTA security measures allow access to personnel data on a "need-to-know" basis. Employees have read-only access to their own data and can check it for accuracy and report any errors needing correction. Supervisors can access data about their employees, and clinical directors and the nurse executive can access employee data across the service.

CLINICAL MODULES

The clinical modules facilitate the processing and improvement of the quality of information used in the provision of patient care. The nursing segment of the electronic clinical record is one component of the hospital clinical information infrastructure. Clinical information nursing systems present the potential for improving nursing diagnosis, care planning and delivery, and patient outcomes. This technology provides for improvement of the quality and availability of clinical data, which is displayed in a more usable format. The clinical nursing software contains modules that address patient assessment, care planning, critical pathways and clinical guidelines, and documentation of physiological parameters. All of these software modules use file structures that promote data integration and transdisciplinary access and use of the total system.

Patient Assessment. Nurses have been the driving force behind the appointment of an interdisciplinary task group made up of nurses, physicians, social workers, respiratory therapists, chaplains, physical and occupational therapists, and dieticians to define specifications for assessment software. The assessment module allows for the collection of data at the lowest level of abstraction. Real-time nursing documentation and retrieval can be realized. Patient assessment, developed in a "Windows"-style environment, uses a graphical user interface (GUI) that can be accessed through the VISTA Nursing Menu. The generic assessment module allows all clinicians to utilize the same tool to collect required assessment data. This capability eliminates redundancies and is more patient-centered. Risk assessment, as a by-product of the generic assessment, has been an added value. A parallel development has been the physician health and physical examination module. The interaction between the two design groups has enhanced the comprehensive nature of both products.

Plan of Care/Clinical Guidelines/Critical Pathways. The database for the care planning module interfaces with the assessment tool. The Care Plan is based on the problem(s) identified through the assessment process. Nurses creating care plans only need to select the most appropriate choices. Module screens cascade through a taxonomic structure of nursing diagnoses, body systems, and/or medical diagnoses. Goals and evaluation dates are established, and interventions appropriate to patient needs are listed. Problems identified as high risk have specific plans of action to produce desired patient outcomes. The flexibility of this module includes the capability for generating guidelines for care of patients with specific nursing diagnoses using the NANDA taxonomy or for specific medical diagnoses that are related to DRG/ICD9 coding. Standardized care guidelines developed by nursing and interdisciplinary experts for specific nursing and/or medical diagnoses are included in the module. The module is flexible enough to allow for the addition of site- or user-specific plans of care.

The field release of care plan software resulted in several creative applications. Some sites used the software exactly as released to produce individualized nursing care plans. Other sites have used the customizing features of this software to build location-specific standards of care and practice. Certain sites used the features of care plan customization to develop interdisciplinary plans of care. The original nursing care plan software is now the conceptual basis of the critical pathway software development. This software module will not contain the clinical content for a pathway but will include a template for local pathway development that can be customized to meet local community standards and unique patient needs. Specifications for this software have been developed by an interdisciplinary task group. The requirements include elements that make its use appropriate in both ambulatory and inpatient care settings. The pathway software will have variance tracking and the ability to generate progress notes that explain these variances.

One by-product of the care planning software is the ability to print a brief or a complete assignment sheet for a patient. This sheet includes specific orders for daily nursing care as well as the planned nursing interventions. The assignment sheet feature has been very positively received by JCAHO. The staff assignment sheet has patient-specific demographic information, diagnosis, and required interventions related to current goals. An end-of-shift summary can also be generated.

Physiological Parameters. Patient vital measurements including temperature, pulse, respiration, weight, central venous pressures, pulse oximetry, and intake and output are examples of the parameters included in the electronic documentation of patient monitoring. The vital signs measurement module, originally developed by nursing, is now utilized by multiple disciplines. The intake/output module stores information regarding amount and type of intake and the amount and type of output for an episode of care. This software interfaces with the intravenous (IV) software in the VISTA Pharmacy application. Patient allergy and/or adverse reaction status is another parameter captured in the VISTA system and available to all treating clinicians.

Treatment Record. An interdisciplinary task group has developed specifications for an automated Treatment Record. This module allows documentation of the date, time, and specific treatments done for both inpatients and outpatients. This software is linked to assessment, care planning, and other VISTA software modules and developed in a GUI format. Treatment Record links directly with OE/RR to extract treatment orders. Again, nurses have been instrumental in this software development.

Progress Notes. The VISTA clinical system has an option for writing narrative notes. All clinicians on the treatment team contribute to the progress notes database and can access notes written for any specific patient. Some sites have chosen to facilitate nursing documentation through the interface of VISTA with commercially developed nursing documentation packages. Nurses document on all aspects of clinical care and may refer to an extensive on-line data dictionary of terms and phrases to structure complete sentences that describe the patient's response to nursing interventions.

Future versions of progress notes will utilize the Text Generator utility, which can be used to build text from codified documents. The end user can make specific selections about the codified data to be used for generation of progress notes text. Currently, the Text Generator is used to create plans of care from selection lists.

Order Entry/Results Reporting (OE/RR). In the progressive movement to an electronic clinical record, highest priority has been given to software applications that integrate clinical patient data. This effort has already begun to cut across hospital services and VISTA software modules. This OE/RR software provides an order format for clinician order entry with functionality that includes an electronic signature, notifications, alerts, and the ability to select individual or team patient lists for action. OE/RR links to the Health Summary module and allows the selection of specific components of health care information such as clinic schedules, clinical laboratory reports, radiology reports, pharmacy profiles, and other patient-specific data to be collected for a consolidated report. This on-line ability eliminates the frantic search for a paper chart if a patient appears in the clinic for care on an unscheduled basis. The information gathered can be provider-, clinic-, or unit-specific. OE/RR is linked to progress notes, the discharge summary, problem list, and clinical lexicon. The problem list allows a provider to enter and retrieve problems/diagnoses. The problem list provides a current and historical view of a patient's problems, and each problem can be traced in terms of treatment, test results, and outcomes. The use of a standardized coding system and cross-referencing of problems, clinical interventions, and patient outcomes is possible. The lexicon maps clinical terminology for NANDA (North American Nursing Diagnosis Association), NIC (Nursing Intervention Classification), the Omaha Nursing System, the International Class of Diseases, and Current Procedural Terminology (CPT) as well as other standard coding systems like ICD9 and *DSM*.

Another module linked to OE/RR is the Consult/Request Tracking module. Consults and procedures can be ordered on-line, and the status of such orders can be tracked and updated. The current discharge summary makes transcribed summaries available on-line, but future plans for this package include the development of a semiautomated summary in which content is derived from the existing electronic record, consolidated, and then presented to the clinician for completion. OE/RR is also linked to vitals measurements, progress notes, allergy/adverse reaction, discharge summary, and the clinical lexicon.

Medication Administration. Pharmacy software modules were designed to increase drug accountability throughout the entire VHA health care system. The Pharmacy modules in VISTA support the frequent interactions between Pharmacy and Nursing Departments regarding inpatient medication administration and the management of controlled substances. Computer-generated Medication Administration Records (MARs) are used to document medications given. MARs can be printed in formats appropriate to specific patient populations. Acute care units with frequent medication changes and the shortest lengths of stay use 24-hour MARs; 7- and 14-day MARs are used on units with longer lengths of stay and less frequent medication adjustments. This module reads from the patient's vitals/measurements and adverse reaction tracking files and automatically prints this information on each MAR. The functionality of the controlled substance module includes monitoring and tracking of the receipt, inventory, and dispensing of all controlled substances. This permits automatic identification of discrepancies and also maintains a perpetual unit/hospital inventory of controlled substances. This functionality has been adapted for use with bar-code technology and hand-held radio-frequency devices that document administration of controlled substances. This technology allows immediate point-of-care computerized documentation of the patient, the medication administered, the nurse giving the medication, and the time.

Patient education sheets are available through the Pharmacy package and can be printed in Spanish or English at several different reading levels. These information sheets are used by both Nursing and Pharmacy to educate patients and their families about ordered medications.

HOSPITAL MANAGEMENT MODULES

Nursing service also uses other VISTA modules that support management functions. These include communication systems, personnel accounting, patient data exchange, and decision support.

"PAID": Personnel and Accounting Integrated Data. The automation of time-keeping and payroll processes now provides nursing administration with "real-time" cost information; hours paid, earned time off, leave usage, overtime, holiday costs, and differential costs for weekend and off-tour staffing. This module is used across all services and has been invaluable in the budgetary process. Computerization of timekeeping has increased accuracy and efficiency and decreased timekeeper work requirements and work hours. The integration of fiscal data with unit census and acuity data can produce reports on costs and nursing hours per patient day. PAID permits employee read-only access to review personal leave balances, check time card accuracy, and request leave. This feature has significantly reduced the paper flow previously necessary to manage time and attendance. Information collection, processing, retrieval, and analysis have been enhanced by computerization. System flexibility allows the production of reports in formats that meet local, regional, and national standards.

Decision Support System (DSS). The extracting and "roll up" of service-specific medical center data into regional and national repositories to aggregate and analyze information is becoming a fiscal necessity. DSS is a commercial state-of-the-art software program designed to extract data that will support an outcomes-oriented method of performance evaluation and improvement. It is being used by the VHA as an enhanced cost accounting system that provides information associated with each episode of care, including nursing care. The software supports longitudinal data collection and analysis and it provides information that allows managers and clinicians to evaluate not only the cost of VHA care, but the quality of care provided to its customers. DSS is being implemented throughout the entire VHA organization over a given time frame.

Electronic Mail. A DHCP package widely utilized by nurses on both a local and a national basis for administrative and clinical communication is the electronic mail system know locally as "Mailman" and nationally as "Forum." The widespread use of e-mail has actually promoted computer literacy among various levels of staff. E-mail is used to create and distribute minutes, maintain task group communication, and in some sites is the easily accessible repository for policies and procedures. Currently, more than 30,000 users are registered in the national "Forum" system.

Patient Data Exchange (PDX). The Patient Data Exchange is an application that has the capability of electronically transferring predefined segments of a patient's medical record between VHA medical centers. This information includes, but is not limited to, the patient's demographics, episodes of care, medications, vital signs, current orders, clinical warnings or crisis notes, progress notes, and diagnostic evaluations. When data arrive at the requesting facility, a mail message is automatically sent notifying the providers that the patient's information has been received from a specific medical center. Once this information is transferred, it can be merged with the patient's pertinent local information. The composite electronic medical record is made available to clinical and administrative staff. The PDX uses the List Manager software that provides screens displaying a list of medical record items from which the user can browse through a cascading array of related patient information. Although the PDX is an initial step in messaging patient data from one facility to another, it is a critical element in providing appropriate interfacility patient services across the continuum of care.

Local Hospital and Areawide Intrafacility Networks. The VHA has established area networks to provide user access to shared directories located at specific domains. Documents residing on these directories contain nursing policies, position papers, committee minutes, user and training manuals, software, and other information that may be shared among VA facilities. Access to directories may be restricted, depending upon the sensitivity of the information or type of directory established. The availability of this network platform promotes transorganizational and organizational communication, decreases infrastructure expenditures, and redirects work flow to promote efficient use of personnel resources.

Department of Veterans Affairs Web Page Access. In 1996, the DVA began using the World Wide Web as a creative approach to provide their clients with current information on VA benefits, health care, and general announcements and methods for addressing concerns and questions on the DVA Home Page. Subsequent information on the Web page also addressed topics of interest in the area of VA research, women veterans' issues, medical automation, patient health information, informatics standards, government resources, AIDS, access to government publications, legislation, testimony, and other government issues. Access to this environment has become so popular that the VA Web Server is rated among the top 5% of all sites on the Internet as stated by POINT SURVEY (DVA Home Page, http://www.va.gov, June, 1996).

The Internet provides nurses with access to the National Library of Medicine and other national libraries and allows direct search on such systems as Medline Current, Medline Previous, CINAHL, and Embase Psychiatry. This capability allows VA nurses to access and integrate current clinical information into daily practice.

EDUCATION TRACKING MODULE

The PAID Education Tracking module was originally designed by nurse educators to be used by VA nursing education. The software is now a generic package that is used by all services throughout the medical centers. All training requests and documentation of attendance at educational programs is done on-line. The education module has enhanced the accuracy of record keeping. Mandatory educational requirements and continuing education for license renewal can be monitored on an ongoing basis by both the employee and the supervisor. Multiple reports can be generated, such as exception reports of personnel who have not completed mandatory training requirements, or the dates mandatory sessions are due.

Maintaining and monitoring the competency of nursing staff has been one of the priority standards for JCAHO. The VISTA education tracking software documents training data for each nursing employee and has been invaluable in supporting the VHA's capability to meet this standard. The nursing application links with the education tracking software and generates education reports by nursing unit. The variety of print options for report generation addresses both local and national requirements. A 3-year cumulative training report per JCAHO requirement can be easily generated. Management of the education budget and equity of support for employee training can be tracked by the number of hours granted or authorized an employee for educational purposes. The number of dollars provided an individual for training is also immediately available for review. The flexibility in defining the various elements that are tracked with definitive time lines are unique aspects of the software. The efficiency of tracking training data and producing customized reports that would take hours to summarize manually saves time, which can be translated into dollar savings. Employees may print their own listing of classes attended and total class hours to ensure mandatory requirements are met and for use in documentation of continuing education for recertification.

National training initiatives mandated for all employees on topics such as "Sexual Harassment" and "Customer Satisfaction" can be tracked by printing the facility attendance lists or deficiency reports. Deficiency reports are electronically generated for any of the mandatory training. The percentage of compliance with training requirements for an individual service or the entire medical center is included in the print options.

Training reports are secured; that is, access to training reports is defined by an individual's position. Employees may access only their own files on a "read/print only" basis, whereas nurse managers have access to files of their unit employees, clinical directors may access section files, and the executive nurse administrator has access to all nursing employees' training files.

END USER SYSTEM TRAINING

Nurses in the VHA health care system must have a working knowledge of VISTA. The Nursing EP has identified training as a high priority in the implementation phase of all new software. The Training Expert Panel has assumed major responsibility for designing educational material for use at all VA centers. National training packages have been developed to assist nurses in using the software and in developing an appreciation of the functionality of the system.

The implementation of the DHCP nursing information system in the multifacility health care settings of the VHA has required a well-defined strategic plan. The plan incorporates policy requirements, leadership designations, and training initiatives. A planned change model has guided the development of strategic education plans for all phases of software implementation. The change agent concept has been operational through the designation of a facilitator training position. Persons given this role are referred to as a Nursing Informatics Coordinator, Clinical Automated Information Support (CAIS) Coordinator, or Automated Data Processing (ADP) Coordinator. The basic functions of this role have been standardized nationally across medical centers. Other functions of persons in these positions may be tailored to the needs of the specific medical centers.

Nursing informatics coordinators have the major responsibility for training nursing employees in the use of the information system. The educational preparation of coordinators varies. Although the initial nursing ADP coordinators received on-the-job training to prepare them for their role, the current required preparation is an advanced degree in Nursing Informatics. In-service training supported from a national budget and implemented through Regional Education Centers prepared the coordinators for specific aspects of the role. Training curriculums encompass such topics as specific functionality for each of the software modules for which the coordinators will be providing instruction, data management, and transfer of information from the mainframe to a PC networked environment. Specifically, the coordinators have support while they learn the role, which includes access to a preceptor/mentor for a designated period of time. Local training may include the acquisition of skills in troubleshooting hardware as well as monitoring of software usage.

The coordinator's responsibility at the local VA site includes designing an implementation manual utilizing material from the national documentation manuals that accompany each software module. Other training materials include basic computer capability with an emphasis on electronic mail as a positive stimulus for learning to use the computer. Nurses in this role may be expected to provide training and coordination for other packages used by nurses, such as order entry, clinical laboratory, dietary, social work, and health summary.

System training has been identified as a planning variable. VA nurses have identified the quality and quantity of planning prior to system implementation as major factors influencing diffusion and adoption of information systems. Abla (1995) identified elements critical to an effective training program as the target population, instructional content, types of instructions, learning environment, and the time allocated for training. Other researchers have provided guidance through the identification of essential skills and knowledge, such as accessing menu driven programs, use of a password, knowledge of entry and retrieval information, security and confidentiality of data, legal issues, and patient rights. Also identified are nonessential skills for the practicing nurse, such as use of a word processor; input/output operations; technical concepts such as Random Access Memory (RAM), Read Only Memory (ROM), and the use of modems; and basic operation of the computer. Inadequate training has been shown to lead to underutilization of software applications and poor user acceptance. The importance of training cannot be overemphasized.

Training laboratories are available at each medical center. The coordinator may have a laboratory with 9 or 10 terminals that allow hands-on experience for learners. These laboratories have microcomputers, software, and access to the hospital computer system through terminal emulations with technology that allows a large display of computer screen images. The training laboratory participants have the opportunity to learn how to utilize software in a safe, supervised environment, where they can become proficient using the applications and understanding the functionality. The training facility also allows coordinators to test new software in a training account before loading into the "live" system.

To expand their capacity for training, coordinators have identified facilitators in each of the nursing units. Nurses in the facilitator roles are volunteers who have demonstrated a special interest and excitement about using computers. The facilitators are accessible to all nursing staff for review of material presented in the training laboratory. This peer-to-peer exchange has increased the comfort of new nurse users and influenced the acceptance of the nursing systems. Adaskin, Hughes, McMullan, McLean, and McMorris (1994) supported this approach in their suggestion about the use of computer preceptors. The quality of training has been the one single variable identified as a factor contributing to user satisfaction with the software.

A challenge that has no specific standard approach for training is preparation for the use of commercial software that supplements VISTA applications. The most frequently used commercial software programs are intensive care unit (ICU) monitoring systems and intelligent staff schedulers. ICU monitoring systems require the coordinator's support of clinicians in the configuration of ICU flow sheets, standardized documentation, and the transfer of selected patient data between the two systems. The implementation of staff schedulers requires extensive work in defining local scheduling rules and practices and in developing appropriate rule-based structures and files in the scheduler to produce computerized schedules acceptable to staff.

The coordinators have responsibility for receiving feedback from end users regarding the benefits of the software in improving efficiency, supporting patient care, and facilitating effective management practices. The system used for communicating desired software enhancements identified at the local facility to national developers is the use of an Enhanced Electronic Error Reporting System (E3R) that communicates recommendations to the development center that produced the software.

POSTIMPLEMENTATION

A significant quantity of nursing time is consumed managing information. Computers collect, store, and transport information in a more efficient way than a manual system. Hence, computers reduce the amount of time required to manage nursing- and patient-specific information, promote cost saving, and support nurse job satisfaction. However, results of research studies of nurses' attitudes toward the use of nursing information systems have been mixed, some positive and others negative (Sultana, 1990). The assessment of attitudes has provided information for the planning and design of educational programs to instruct nurses in the use of computers in health care settings.

Despite all of the planning and training for the VA Nursing Information System, a survey of medical centers showed variations in the usage of the available VISTA software. Nurse application coordinators functioned as facilitators in a survey of VISTA package usage throughout the VHA medical centers. Questions focused on the identification of all VISTA software used at a medical center. Clinical packages with the greatest percentage of use included patient classification (98.4%), clinical laboratory (97.1%), radiology (96.1%), social work (91.1%), and dietetics (96.7%). The most widely used clinical packages are those that relate to the flow of information between the nursing units and other ancillary departments. These applications have been found to save time for nurses and result in frequent use (Hendrickson & Kovner, 1990). The packages with lower use rates included patient care plans (54.7%) and vitals measurements (17.5%; see Figure 11.3). Limited implementation of these clinical packages seems related to the need for point-of-care technology for greater user acceptance; for example, workstations or portable entry devices on the nursing units. The administrative packages with the highest percentage of use included PAID, the national mandated fiscal payroll software (100%), bed control (92%), and inpatient list and incident reporting (95%; Department of Veterans Affairs, Veterans Health Administration, 1996; see Figure 11.4).

Although the VHA has identified the development of clinical applications as its highest priority for computerization, this position has not been consistently reflected in the use of available clinical software. Clinicians have been the most difficult group to convince of the value of incorporating the use of computers in their practice. Nurses may have difficulty accepting computers as adjunct to their decision-making role. Variations in implementation may also be related to workload and the availability of time to attend computer training educational programs. The nurse having the higher level of computer competence will also have a higher level of comfort in using computers. Studies have indicated that those nurses with a given comfort level found computers added

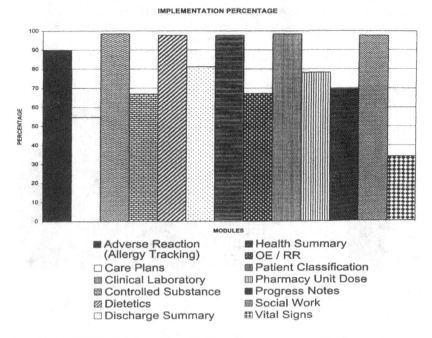

IMPLEMENTATION PERCENTAGE

Adverse Reaction (Allergy Tracking)
□ Care Plans
▧ Clinical Laboratory
▨ Controlled Substance
▨ Dietetics
□ Discharge Summary

■ Health Summary
▨ OE / RR
▨ Patient Classification
▥ Pharmacy Unit Dose
■ Progress Notes
▨ Social Work
▨ Vital Signs

Figure 11.3. VISTA Software Clinical Package Use

excitement to the job (Ngin, Simms, & Erbin-Roesemann, 1993). Developers of clinical packages need to be sensitive to the importance of producing programs that support the actual clinical process used in the delivery of patient care. Ease of use through user-friendly interfaces, graphical screen presentations, and quick access tools such as pointers and light pens may be the controlling variable for implementation of computerized systems and the diffusion of clinical software. The cost and accessibility of hardware for efficient use of systems has also been a variable that influences system acceptance.

Cost Variables. The cost of hardware has been a factor in limiting full utilization of all VISTA software at all VA medical centers. VA nurse executives are expected to have input in the medical center information system plan. The number and type of input devices needed on a nursing unit should be identified by nursing. This requirement subsumes a knowledge base of state-of-the-art computer technology. The VA Nursing Informatics Constituency Center incorporated an example of a Nursing Service ADP Budget Plan in their report of software usage and needs. A modified sizing model approach was used in defining requirements. The bed capacity and number of users were primary variables dictating

ADMINISTRATIVE MODULE

IMPLEMENTATION PERCENTAGE

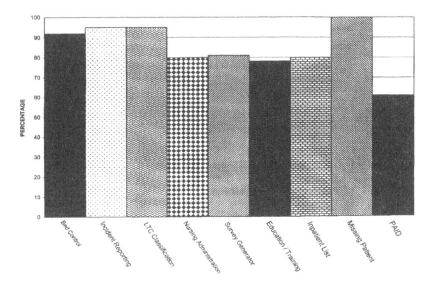

Figure 11.4. VISTA Software Administrative Package Use

quantity of hardware (Department of Veterans Affairs, Veterans Health Administration, 1996).

Training cost was also found to be a factor influencing full implementation. Computer assisted instruction and computer assisted learning should be nurtured because of their cost-effectiveness. Learning realized with the help of a computer and no direct interaction of the user with a human instructor is a self-directed learning approach that has been credited with greater knowledge retention, enhanced clinical judgment, and less instruction time in comparison to more traditional teaching methods (Nerlich, 1995). Using adult learning principles and curriculum design concepts to develop these programs for nurses in direct clinical roles should ensure greater acceptance and use of information systems by nurses.

Point of Care. One common thread that prevents the investiture of an automated medical record from becoming a reality is the lack of a point-of-care environment. Over the past several years, the VHA has begun to address the need for a fiber-optic backbone. The backbone is used to support the hardware that clinicians require to enter assessments, record treatments, document patient education, access clinical decision support-based applications, and collect other relevant patient information. Clinical care environments must be designed and constructed with clinical computing and telenursing as the basis for providing high-quality patient care. Workstations and lightweight portable hand-held terminals that utilize wireless LANs will be the minimal standard requirements acceptable throughout all medical care facilities, including extended care.

FUTURE INITIATIVES

The use of more sophisticated hardware such as wireless systems, voice technology, and real-time telecommunications figures prominently in the future of the VHA. World Wide Web technology will provide clinicians with quick access to patient information from within the VHA health system network. Telephone triage using interactive voice response systems for scheduling appointments, obtaining patient health information, and requesting refills of prescriptions are only a few of the conveniences that the agency will offer patients to facilitate access to care and enhance patient satisfaction with the VHA health care system.

The distribution of diagnostic test results to clinicians through clinical imaging systems, on-line data retrieval of EKG tracing graphics, and telepathology using high resolution techniques and robotics will become an inherent part of health care facilities. The patient in a remote location can benefit from expert on-line diagnostic evaluation. Robotics is already in wide use for Pathology and Radiology Departments. VHA regional and national database repositories will be established to support clinical research, to trend care, and to share patient information among hospitals, providers, and patients. VHA and Department of Defense sharing activities will increase, and the combined services provided to patients will be seamless. Links between the VHA data systems and other federal health care programs (e.g., Medicare and Medicaid) will be established.

Clinical Expert Decision Support Systems. The primary focus of this hospital information system has shifted from administrative applications to clinical applications. The VISTA software has laid a foundation for clinical decision support. Currently, application developers have provided software checks in specific DHCP software packages (e.g., Adverse Reaction, Plans of Care, Clinical Guidelines, Vitals/Measurements, and Order Entry/Results Reporting) that provide a limited automated decision support system. The patient database provides an environment-rich repository of information used to assist clinicians in the planning and delivery of patient care. Additional application development, however, is required in the area of physician-based history and physical examinations, encoding of patient data, vendor interface standards, and artificial intelligence, before extensive clinical decision support can be fully realized.

Nursing software modules have become an integral part of the entire VHA health care information infrastructure. VHA nursing has made a major contribution to the identification and capture of the elements of nursing practice that contribute to patient care outcomes. External database linkages are being maintained for the purpose of sharing and comparing patient information across systems and supporting nursing research. Analysis of this data provides the opportunity for continuous improvement of the quality of care delivered. Nursing will continue to have a role in the ongoing development of the Veterans Health Information Systems Technology Architecture.

NOTE

1. This information is from a verbal report given in May 1996 by J. Dietrich, Freedom of Information Act Coordinator, Hines Information Resource Management Field Office, Hines, IL.

REFERENCES

Abla, S. (1995). The who, what, where, when, and how of computer education. *Computers in Nursing, 13*(3), 114-117.

Adaskin, E., Hughes, L., McMullan, P., McLean, M., & McMorris, D. (1994). The impact of computerization in nursing: An interview study of users and facilitators. *Computers in Nursing, 12*(3), 141-148.

Ball, S. (1994). Defining information management requirements. In K. Hannah, M. Ball, & M. Edwards (Eds.), *Introduction to nursing informatics* (chap. 3). New York: Springer.

Department of Veterans Affairs. (1995). *Veterans Health Administration annual report.* Washington, DC: Author.

Department of Veterans Affairs, Veterans Health Administration. (1995). *Decentralized hospital computer program* (Medical Information Resources Management Office). Washington, DC: Author.

Department of Veterans Affairs, Veterans Health Administration. (1996). *Informatics Constituency Center report.* Unpublished report, VHA Nursing Service, Washington, DC.

Department of Veterans Affairs Home Page. (1996, June). Available: http://www.va.gov.

Hendrickson, G., & Kovner, C. (1990). Effects of computers on nursing resource use: Do computers save nurses time? *Computers in Nursing, 8*(1), 16-22.

Lewkowicz, J. (1989). *The complete MUMPS: An introduction and reference for the MUMPS programming language* (pp. 1-3). Englewood Cliffs, NJ: Prentice Hall.

Nerlich, S. (1995). Computer assisted learning (CAL) for general and specialist nursing education. *Australian Critical Care, 8*(3), 23-27.

Ngin, P., Simms, L., & Erbin-Roesemann, M. (1993). Work excitement among computer users in nursing. *Computers in Nursing, 11*(3), 127-133.

Sultana, N. (1990). Nurses' attitudes toward computerization in clinical practice. *Computers in Nursing, 13*(3), 118-121.

CHAPTER 12

A Case Study in Cost-Effectiveness Analysis for Computer Technology Used in Support of Caregivers With Alzheimer's Disease Patients

Russell C. McGuire

Two areas of concern associated with providing in-home care to patients with Alzheimer's disease are social isolation and difficulty in receiving information to support decision making by the caregiver. Patricia Brennan, PhD, and her colleagues demonstrated the effectiveness of a computer system known as ComputerLink in reducing caregivers' social isolation and increasing their decision-making confidence. This case study demonstrates the simplicity of using an economic analysis such as cost-effectiveness for determining the worth of this technology within a particular health care delivery system.

The case study reported here is a cost-effectiveness analysis of decision support based on caregiver decision confidence scores in both an experimental and a control group. The cost-effectiveness ratios demonstrated that when all three elements of the ComputerLink system were used in support of caregiver decision making, the system was more cost-effective than traditional support methods.

Delivery of health care in the United States is a continuous challenge in the allocation of limited resources. The current response to this challenge is to reengineer the delivery of health care to decrease inpatient utilization. More home care use is being used in all regions of the nation. Along with this increased reliance upon home care is the need for increased support for caregivers isolated within the home environment.

Caregivers of Alzheimer's patients face daily challenges in providing care to these patients. These challenges include the need for acquiring relevant information, coping with unforeseen problems associated with caregiving, reducing social isolation, and establishing and maintaining both social support and decision-making support (Brennan, Moore, & Smyth, 1991). Demands on the caregiver range from simple (e.g., assisting the Alzheimer's disease [AD] patient with dressing) to complex (e.g., dealing with the severe behavioral and physical problems experienced during the later phases of the disease process). Caregiver time and resource use increase as the complexity of the disease progresses. As caregiver burden increases, there is often a resultant increase in social isolation, anxiety, and physical fatigue. Support mechanisms may not be readily accessible to the caregiver due to time constraints and financial costs associated with the caregiving situation. With increased burden, caregivers of Alzheimer's patients require an effective and low-cost means of in-home support. Interventions providing caregiver education, reduction in social isolation, and decision-making support are necessary for relieving the stress associated with caregiving.

Brennan and colleagues (1991) demonstrated that caregivers of Alzheimer's patients can benefit from the use of automated computer technology, based upon nursing interventions, by providing "physical, emotional, and environmental support for their loved ones" (p. 15). Through the use of a computer network known as ComputerLink, an electronic encyclopedia, an automated decision support system, and electronic communications are available to caregivers of Alzheimer's patients in their home settings (Brennan, 1994).

The electronic encyclopedia provides information about Alzheimer's disease, caregiving strategies, clinical care of the Alzheimer's patient, and a reference of local services. The decision support system uses a technique known as "decision modeling," which is the core of the decision support element of ComputerLink. Decision modeling uses the existing knowledge of the caregiver and guides the caregiver in the selection of alternative solutions for caregiving challenges based upon the caregiver's beliefs and values. The electronic communications segment provides access to both peers and professional caregivers. Caregivers participated in an electronic public forum, sent and received electronic mail, and asked questions in anonymity that were answered by a project nurse. The project team consisted of five nurses, a sociologist, and a psychologist who developed the content and created the network.

Brennan (1994) and her colleagues demonstrated that ComputerLink effectively reduced social isolation, increased communication, increased caregiver knowledge, and increased caregiver decision-making confidence. While Brennan's work demonstrated the effectiveness of this technology in meeting caregiver's needs, the relative cost-effectiveness of ComputerLink in comparison with more traditional forms of support and sources of information was not addressed. Understanding the cost-effectiveness of alternative modes for nursing interventions is critical for nurse executives who must make decisions about optimal resource allocation.

HISTORICAL PERSPECTIVE

In a randomized study, decision-making skills, perception of social isolation, and physical health status of Alzheimer's caregivers were studied (Brennan et al., 1991). A convenience sample of caregivers of Alzheimer's patients was identified from an Alzheimer's disease research registry established with a university-affiliated hospital in the Cleveland, Ohio, area. An experimental group consisting of caregivers of Alzheimer's patients was randomly selected, and computer equipment consisting of a video terminal (WYSE 30), a keyboard, and a 1,200 baud modem were installed in the homes of the caregivers. Training on this equipment was provided in a 1.5 hour session, conducted by one of the project nurses. The training consisted of explanations and demonstrations of the network components, a return demonstration, and a written instructional pamphlet. A control group of caregivers of Alzheimer's patients received a monthly telephone call as a placebo intervention. A passive electronic monitoring system was used to collect information continuously regarding the caregivers' use of the various components of the system as users logged on to the system.

As the study began to provide more data related to the extent of Computer-Link use by the caregivers, Brennan was able to document evidence that the technology supported insightful, supportive communications between the caregiver and the health care professional. The trend in the use of the technology continued to demonstrate that communication functions were used the most often, followed by the electronic encyclopedia and the decision support elements.

Continued data collection demonstrated use of the decision support element to resolve questions related to placement of an Alzheimer's patient in a nursing home, communication with co-caregivers, and choice of where a caregiver should live with an Alzheimer's patient. Brennan found that ComputerLink use fostered communication in a less inhibited and more assertive manner. Open communication among participants appeared to be more intimate than face-to-face communication. These findings supported earlier research related to the use of decision support systems (Brennan, 1986, 1987; Brennan & McHugh, 1988; Hannah, 1988; Ozbolt, 1988).

DECISION SUPPORT

A decision support system (DSS) is an automated system that capitalizes on the skills of the user and the computer to solve problems that neither the computer nor user could solve alone. A DSS is used to supplement or augment the problem-solving skills of the user, whether the user is a skilled health care professional or a health care recipient. System components may vary from user to user; that is, what constitutes a DSS for a particular user facing a specific problem may not be the same for another user facing the same problem (Brennan, 1987). Essential components include (a) a complete software solution to assist the user in making complex decisions and (b) contributions by both the user and the computer to the decision-making process. Expected user outcomes for DSS use should include (a) substantial reduction in decision-making time, (b) access to a large database of information, (c) the ability to "conceptualize" the entire scope of the problem, and (d) assisted mobility through the problem-solving process (Brennan & McHugh, 1988, p. 91).

COST ANALYSIS AND INFORMATIONAL TECHNOLOGY

Very little has been written about the cost-effectiveness of computer use in nursing, although it is estimated that the use of economic analysis increased 50-fold between 1966 and 1990 (Gilbaldi & Sullivan, 1994). The ever-increasing need to justify new health care programs and technologies has both federal government and private sector health care payers searching for methods to assist in making informed decisions regarding medical technology costs. Commonly used approaches include cost-effectiveness analysis, cost utility, and cost-benefit approaches. Of these, cost-effectiveness analysis is superior because of its ability to account for both quantitative and qualitative data while analyzing alternative interventions (Hannah, 1988).

A cost-effectiveness ratio is the measurement of incremental cost (i.e., the difference in cost between the original intervention and the alternative) and the intervention's effectiveness in achieving a predetermined goal (Hannah, 1988). These ratios are compared to a predetermined cut-off. An intervention whose ratio is greater than the cut-off is deemed unacceptable. Ratios must be established for each of the alternatives under consideration (Hannah, 1988). These ratios are compared in the formula

$$GE1/C1 > GE2/C2$$

where GE equals measures of goal effectiveness and C equals costs.

Cost analysis requires a comparison of benefits gained versus resources utilized and should be used in conjunction with other appropriate assessments of a project's worth to the community. Otherwise, health care payers could inadvertently circumvent the justified intentions of health care providers and "discard an expensive intervention that provides substantial benefit in favor of an inexpensive one that provides an important but more modest, less dramatic or less immediate benefit" (Gilbaldi & Sullivan, 1994, p. 411).

A carefully designed research approach that includes a randomized selection process and tight control of the study is essential (Garber, 1994). Researchers face many difficulties inherent in the various cost-effectiveness analysis methods available (Neumann & Johannesson, 1994). Data availability and data sources may add bias to a cost-effectiveness study. The rapid rate of change in technological advances often makes it difficult to adequately compare "replacement" technology to "existing" technology. Various design variables must also be considered. A number of analysis methods are available to researchers, and many differ in both the definition and the measurement of cost. Present value versus future value and benefit are difficult to assess along a constantly advancing time continuum. Accurate discounted costs may be affected by the use of varying levels of discounting rates by different researchers.

ANALYTICAL METHOD

The method used for this study is cost-effectiveness analysis (Levin, 1983). The research design used for this study was a secondary data analysis using Brennan's research comparing computer support with traditional methods of support for caregivers of people with Alzheimer's. Brennan randomly selected participants in the experimental and control groups for her Alzheimer's caregiver study. Cost data from the experimental group (users of ComputerLink) were compared with those of the control group. The variables identified for this cost-effectiveness analysis were the costs associated with providing support and care to caregivers of Alzheimer's patients in the home setting and the relationship of these costs to caregiver decision confidence.

INSTRUMENTATION

A cost estimation table was used to identify and categorize total project costs (see Table 12.1, below). The Ingredient list was taken from Brennan's (U.S. Public Health Service, 1990, R01-AG08617-13) original Computerlink budget projection and includes all components of resource utilization—personnel, facilities, materials, equipment, and caregivers' time. Initial start-up costs for development, purchase, and maintenance of software and hardware is also included.

Total Costs lists the total summed value of all resources used. Allocation of these costs to either sponsor or caregiver is also identified. Caregiver Costs include any costs incurred directly by the caregiver/patient that were not covered in the specific project ingredient list, such as home environment modification.

ComputerLink Project Costs Estimations

The estimated costs for the ComputerLink project were identified from Brennan's (1990) first-year project cost projections. The following cost categories were used: equipment, personnel, utility (e.g., electricity), caregiver costs, network modification and maintenance, office supplies, consultants, travel, photocopying/communication, and computer time. The costs for the experimental group ($N = 47$) were identified and assigned to the "total ingredient cost" and to the appropriate subcategories. The majority of the costs were identified and assigned to the "costs to sponsor" subcategory, which in this case was the National Institute on Aging and the National Institute of Health. The only other subcategory costs identified were associated with "caregiver imposed cost." No costs were identified for other government and/or community sources or for contributed private inputs. Nonmonetary costs, such as caregiver burden, were not included in the experimental or control group cost estimations due to lack of verifiable data. Nevertheless, nonmonetary costs can have an impact on the cost-effectiveness of a particular project. Using Levin's (1983) criteria for categorizing costs associated with a project, caregiver burden would have been placed in the category "costs imposed to caregivers." Costs associated with caregiver burden could be reflected in varying levels of caregiver stress and the medical costs for coping with these stressors. Cost per ComputerLink use (Ccl) was computed by dividing the total net project cost by the total number of ComputerLink log-ons.

Cost Estimation for
Experimental and Control Groups

Service contact data for the experimental and control groups were gathered at Case Western Reserve University and, for the purpose of comparison, equate to the use of the ComputerLink components for support of caregiver decision making. The service contact data were collected for the experimental and control groups through monthly telephone contact by the project staff. Estimated cost per service use for both groups was calculated from cost data gathered during a 1976 General Accounting Office study looking at cost of care for the elderly with dementia in the Cleveland, Ohio, area (Mindel, Wright, & Starrett, 1986). The 1976 costs were adjusted to 1990 project year costs by multiplying the original cost by an indexed factor. The indexed factor was calculated by dividing the 1990 Medical Consumer Price Index by the 1976 Medical Consumer Price Index (Finkler, 1992; U.S. Department of Commerce, 1994). The cost adjustment index (see Table 12.4, below) was thus developed by dividing the 1990 Medical Consumer Price Index (MCPI), 162.8, by the 1976 MCPI, 52.0.

This index, 3.13, was multiplied by the 1976 costs associated with the following categories: hospitals visits, medical care (caregiver), medical care (patient), skilled nursing care, support groups, and referral services (Mindel et al., 1986). Total service contacts were totaled and divided into the total 1990 adjusted costs, yielding an average service cost per use for both the experimental and the control groups.

Effectiveness Measurements for
ComputerLink and Control Groups

The elements for this study's cost-effectiveness analysis were taken from the measurement of decision confidence (Brennan, 1995). The original hypothesis for decision support in the Brennan study was that ComputerLink would enhance the decision-making confidence of the AD caregiver. The Brennan study used modification of a decision scale developed by Saunders and Courtney (1986). The original 22-item instrument was shortened to 14 items reflecting decision confidence. Data were collected using an interview format. The interviewer prompted the caregiver to think about a recent important decision and mark the response on a Likert-type scale, ranging from 1 for *strong agreement* to 5 for *strong disagreement*. The items were summed, with the higher scores reflecting a greater decision-making confidence. The resulting scores ranged from 14 to 70. Brennan (1995) reported that the Cronbach's alpha for this instrument was .88 for the sample.

PROCEDURE

Data processing and analysis were performed using net cost calculations and effectiveness measurements for each component of the experimental and control group to develop the cost-effectiveness ratio. Analysis and comparisons between the experimental and control groups were based upon cost-effectiveness ratios (CE ratio) described by Hannah (1988). The equation establishes a ratio for both the new intervention and the established intervention. A cost-effectiveness equation is used to determine if there are any differences in cost per unit of use (C) and effectiveness (GE) between two groups—in this case, the ComputerLink group (cl) and the control group (c). The traditional cost-effectiveness formula described by Hannah (1988) was modified for this study to identify the specific effectiveness measure chosen, that is, decision confidence (D):

$$\text{Traditional cost-effectiveness formula: } GE1/C1 \geq GE2/C2$$

$$\text{Modified for this study: } Dcl/Ccl \geq Dc/Cc$$

RESULTS

Cost Findings

Costs to the sponsor for the first year of the ComputerLink project were $141,204.00. Total project costs were $141,704.00 with the addition of the caregiver cost. Table 12.1 depicts the costs associated with the experimental group.

The experimental group's use of the system was measured with passive electronic monitoring of logging on to the individual components of the ComputerLink system. Log-ons were measured for the electronic encyclopedia, decision support, forum, and Q&A sections. Table 12.2 shows usage of the different components of the ComputerLink system.

The average cost per user and the allocation of cost per ComputerLink component log-on were calculated by dividing the total project costs, $141,704.00, by the total ComputerLink component usage, 4,333. The average cost per use was calculated as $32.70. The highest average costs per use in

TABLE 12.1   ComputerLink Project Costs (Experimental Group)

Ingredient	Total Costs ($)	Cost to Sponsor ($)	Caregiver Cost ($)
Equipment	22,050.00	22,050.00	
Personnel	93,229.00	93,229.00	
Utilities	3,125.00	3,125.00	
Caregiver cost	500.00		500.00
Network modification and maintenance	10,325.00	10,325.00	
Office supplies	2,275.00	2,275.00	
Consultants	4,300.00	4,300.00	
Travel	2,900.00	2,900.00	
Photocopying and communications	1,500.00	1,500.00	
Computer time	1,000.00	1,000.00	
Total	141,704.00	141,204.00	500.00

TABLE 12.2   ComputerLink Component Usage (Experimental Group)

Component	Use of Component	Percentage Use
Electronic encyclopedia	518	11.95
Decision support	91	2.10
Forum	2,856	65.92
Q&A section	868	20.03
Total	4,333	100.00
Cost per ComputerLink usage	32.70	

SOURCE: McGuire, 1995.

descending order are with the use of the forum, Q&A section, electronic encyclopedia, and decision support.

Further costs for the experimental and control groups were estimated due to lack of available cost data from the Brennan et al. (1991) study. This estimation was made using data gathered during a 1976 Government Accounting Office study looking at the cost associated with the care of elderly people with dementia in the Cleveland, Ohio, area (Mindel et al., 1986). Service contact categories were identified for both the Mindel and the Brennan studies. These categories include hospital visits, medical care for both the caregiver and the patient, skilled nursing care, support groups, and referral services. Each of the service contact entities have potential decision-making support functions for the caregivers. Telephone inquiry was performed by Brennan et al. (1991) to ascertain the number of monthly service contacts for both the experimental and control groups. A comparison of the service contact data between the experimental and control groups shows that the control group had higher

TABLE 12.3 Estimated Service Cost Data for Control and Experimental Groups
(Project Year 1990)

Service Contact	Total Contacts Control	Total Contacts Experimental
Hospital visits	27	22
Medical care, caregiver	117	89
Medical care, patient	118	117
Skilled nursing care	16	24
Support groups	73	84
Referral services	31	40

TABLE 12.4 Inflation Index Factor and Adjusted Cost Formula

Medical Consumer Price Index	Inflation Index Formula
1976 = 52.0	1990 MCPI/1976 MCPI = Index Factor
1990 = 162.8	162.8/52.0 = 3.13

Service Contacts	Estimated 1976 Costs	Adjusted 1990 Costs (1976 costs × index factor)
Hospital visits	128.67	402.84
Medical visits (patient)	12.00	37.57
Medical care (caregiver)	12.00	37.57
Skilled nursing care	23.00	74.83
Support groups	4.32	13.52
Referral services	6.49	20.32

SOURCE: Finkler & Kovner, 1993.

service contact levels for hospital visits (patient), medical care (caregiver), and referral services for both the patient and caregiver. Higher levels of service contact for the experimental group were found for medical care (patient), skilled nursing (patient), and support group use (caregiver).

Total service contacts for the experimental and control groups are summarized in Table 12.3. Both patients and caregivers used medical care services more often than any other category. Total service contact for the project year was 382 contacts for the control group and 376 for the experimental group.

Cost estimations for each of the service contact categories were performed using the Mindel et al. (1986) data and adjusting the 1976 cost figures to 1990 project year cost figures. The adjustment of the 1976 cost figures was made by calculating an adjustment index from the 1976 and 1990 Medical Consumer Price Indexes. The index equation is demonstrated in Table 12.4.

TABLE 12.5 Cost Adjustment Calculations for the Control Group

Service Contact	Estimated Costs (1976 Dollars)	Adjusted Costs (1990 Dollars)	Total in 1990 Dollars
Hospital visits	128.67	402.84	10,876.57
Medical care (caregiver)	12.00	37.57	4,395.60
Medical care (patient)	12.00	37.57	4,433.17
Skilled nursing care	23.90	74.83	1,197.21
Support groups	4.32	13.52	987.32
Referral services	6.49	20.32	629.88
Total Service Costs: $22,519.75			
Mean Service Costs: $58.70			

TABLE 12.6 Cost Adjustment Calculations for the Experimental Group

Service Contact	Estimated Costs (1976 Dollars)	Adjusted Costs (1990 Dollars)	Total in 1990 Dollars
Hospital visits	128.67	402.84	8,862.48
Medical care (caregiver)	12.00	37.57	3,343.73
Medical care (patient)	12.00	37.57	4,395.69
Skilled nursing care	23.90	74.83	1,795.92
Support groups	4.32	13.52	1,135.68
Referral services	6.49	20.32	812.80
Total Service Costs: $20,346.30			
Mean Service Costs: $54.11			

Tables 12.5 and 12.6 demonstrate the 1976 costs, the cost adjustment index, and the 1990 adjusted costs for each of the service contact categories for the control group and experimental groups, respectively.

The average service cost for the control group is $58.70. This figure is calculated by dividing the total service costs for the control group by the total number of service contacts. The same calculation was made for the experimental group and was added to the ComputerLink average cost per component use.

Effectiveness Findings

The average decision confidence scores for the ComputerLink group and the control group are depicted in Table 12.7. The mean scores for the decision confidence measurement were computed during pretest (Time 1) and posttest (Time 2) periods. The study group mean difference scores were computed and subjected to a t test; the results indicated a significant difference ($t = -2.73$, $p < .01$) in the mean change scores (Brennan, 1995).

TABLE 12.7   Decision Confidence Measurements (Experimental and Control
             Groups)

		Control	Experimental
Decision Confidence	Time 1	54.65	51.90
	Time 2	54.70	56.80
	Difference	0.05**	4.90**

SOURCE: Brennan, Moore, & Smyth, 1995.
** $p \leq 0.01$

TABLE 12.8   Cost-Effectiveness Equation Results (Experimental Versus Control
             Groups)

Dcl = Decision confidence, ComputerLink	4.90
Dc = Decision confidence, Control group	0.05
Ccl = Cost, ComputerLink	$86.81
Ccc = Cost, Control group	$58.70

$$\text{Dcl : Ccl} \geq \text{Dc : Cc}$$
$$4.90 : 86.81 \geq .05 : 58.70$$
$$0.06 \geq 0.001$$

The first cost-effectiveness equation and the results are depicted in Table 12.8. This equation demonstrates that ComputerLink's cost-effectiveness ratio is greater than that of the traditional support methods in providing the caregiver an increase in decision-making confidence.

DISCUSSION

Brennan demonstrated the effective use of ComputerLink and its positive effects on the AD caregiving experience. Reductions in social isolation and increases in decision confidence were demonstrated in the experimental group. The cost-effectiveness of the ComputerLink project versus traditional formal and informal methods of caregiver support is demonstrated in this present study.

ComputerLink Systems Costs

The cost-effectiveness formula shows that the cost of the average use of ComputerLink was greater than the cost of the estimated average service contact use for the control group ($86.81 vs. $58.70). From a clinical perspective, the costs for ComputerLink supporting caregivers' decision making demonstrates this modality's worth as an enhancement in situations where (a) the caregiver is isolated from traditional formal and informal support mechanisms, (b) the time expended for caregiving places demands on the caregiver's schedule, and (c) the system's components are used in conjunction with traditional formal support methods. The cost of providing ComputerLink to reduce caregiver isolation and to support decision-making confidence includes all elements of the system as well as the use of traditional methods of support, and allows for independent caregiver research in a resource-rich computerized environment. This is in contrast to traditional formal and informal support mechanisms where the caregiver must rely on the health care provider's knowledge, and facilities where costs for providing support services are often much higher than the ComputerLink costs. An element of convenience is incorporated into the ComputerLink system. This convenience is demonstrated in the ability of the system to allow the AD caregiver effective access based upon the caregiver's schedule versus that of the health care provider's and support group's. Access to the system is allowed day or night and is not dependent upon real-time health care or social support provider presence. This reduces travel and nonproductive wage loss to the AD caregiver, if the caregiver is seeking elements of education, communication, or decision support that are supported by the system.

This study demonstrates the efficacy of ComputerLink in comparison with the use of traditional formal support systems when caregivers of Alzheimer's patients are in need of support in the decision-making process. One can argue that the experimental group is also exposed to the same influences of contact with formal support systems and thus must also include the costs per service contact with that of the average costs per ComputerLink use. This would then increase the ComputerLink costs and affect the outcome of the cost-effectiveness analysis, and the ComputerLink system then must be viewed as an enhancement used in conjunction with formal support systems.

ComputerLink System Effectiveness

There are many methods available to provide support to caregivers of Alzheimer's patients. These support methods are often provided by institutions such as hospitals, clinics, and community resources. For example, local Alzheimer's disease support groups commonly provide assistance to caregivers. The vast array of support providers can be difficult to identify, as is determining the extent of services offered to the caregiver. Support in the form of communication and validation of the caregiver's decision making is often sought by the caregiver in the form of professional health care and social services provider knowledge. Communications with professional, social services, and AD peer care providers allow the AD caregiver the opportunity to validate decision making, thus enhancing decision-making confidence. Both the traditional support method (monthly telephone follow-up) and ComputerLink provide this support. ComputerLink provides access to elements of the computer system that support decision making, but ComputerLink is more effective in increasing AD caregiver decision-making confidence. This effectiveness is demonstrated by the differences in the Time 1 and Time 2 (pre- and posttest) measurements of the experimental and control groups' decision confidence scores (decision confidence score, ComputerLink = 4.90; decision confidence score, control group = 0.05).

Limitations

Possible limitations to this study include limited data for the control group and the retrospective nature of the cost data. At the time of this analysis, very little cost or service utilization data had been documented in the literature on people with Alzheimer's disease. Since the cost components and effectiveness measurements should be calculated and compared at the same time in the implementation of the ComputerLink project and the traditional methods, variations in the two CE ratio components may have varying degrees of accuracy. If the cost and effectiveness data for the control group are inadequate or nonretrievable, possible substitute comparisons of other formal and informal support methods in the Cleveland, Ohio, area may be used, or appropriate national cost averages used for the control group. Exact figures for large cost components/ingredients such as facilities, utilities, depreciation, and the like, may have varying degrees of accuracy due to difficulty in identifying exact cost composition.

Cost data for the ComputerLink project were documented in the original grant proposal and were used in this study as a baseline for total program cost. Actual costs associated with the Brennan study were not available at the time of analysis for this cost-effectiveness study. While the exact costs associated with the study would enhance the accuracy of the cost-effectiveness analysis, it is believed that the actual costs were reasonably within the projected project cost and thus reflect a fairly accurate cost-effectiveness ratio for the ComputerLink and control groups. If replicated, it would be recommended that a future study include a more extensive and proactive determination of exact costs associated with an individual's caregiving within the home.

Several assumptions must be made regarding the estimated average cost of service contact use for the control group. First, although the cost is used in relation to decision confidence, the estimated cost for service contact is not exclusive of other elements of AD caregiver and health care provider interaction. For example, the estimated cost for the control group would also include service elements such as treatments and diagnostic testing. Limitations on the cost data include a lack of data on the electronic infrastructure that supports ComputerLink. Those costs encompass the expense associated with the operation of the Cleveland FreeNet. These costs were unattainable for this study. The Cleveland FreeNet operation costs constitute an element of total costs associated with the ComputerLink systems operation. Without the Cleveland FreeNet, the ComputerLink systems costs would be underestimated. The Cleveland FreeNet provides the network hardware, software, and systems maintenance that make it possible to utilize ComputerLink.

The effectiveness measure used for this study is only one element of the overall effectiveness of the ComputerLink system. Further identification of systems effectiveness should be considered to determine as completely as possible the cost-effectiveness of the system. An exploration of a cost-effectiveness method encompassing a qualitative measurement of social isolation would help provide a comprehensive evaluation of the cost-effectiveness of ComputerLink.

Finally, it is not clear whether the results of this study can be generalized to other populations. The Brennan study and this cost-effectiveness study are limited to a single population of Alzheimer's disease caregivers in a single city.

CONCLUSIONS

ComputerLink has been successfully used in the homes of caregivers of Alzheimer's disease patients and people with AIDS (PWA). Brennan and her colleagues demonstrated the effectiveness of ComputerLink in reducing social isolation and increasing caregiver decision-making confidence. The study reported here concludes that when all elements of ComputerLink, that is, the electronic encyclopedia, the electronic forum, the question and answer element, and the decision support system, are used by the AD caregiver, ComputerLink is cost-effective.

Suggestions for Future Research

Future considerations for ComputerLink research should include replication of the system's elements in a rural setting. Costs associated with access for the urban caregiver versus those of a rural user will likely be different. Research into the use and the associated cost-effectiveness of home computer support should be replicated in a population that has similar access and caregiver issues. Persons with physical limitations, for example, could benefit from using this technology to guide and assist their rehabilitation efforts.

REFERENCES

Brennan, P. (1986). A meaning behind the BUZZ. *Computers in Nursing, 4*(2), 51, 96.

Brennan, P. (1987). Computerized decision support: Beyond expert systems. *Health Matrix, 5*(2), 31-33.

Brennan, P. (1994). Differential use of computer network services. *Proceedings of the American Medical Informatics Association, Annual Symposium on Computer Applications in Medical Care,* pp. 27-31.

Brennan, P. (1995). *Alzheimer's disease subjects.* Unpublished manuscript. (Available from Russell C. McGuire, Director of Clinical Services, Division of Home Services, Appalachian Regional Healthcare, 100 Airport Gardens-Suite 5, Hazard, KY 41701; rmcgu0@ukcc.uky.edu)

Brennan, P., & McHugh, M. (1988). Clinical decision-making and computer support. *Applied Nursing Research, 1*(2), 89-93.

Brennan, P., Moore, S., & Smyth, K. (1991). ComputerLink: Electronic support for the home caregiver. *Advanced Nursing Science, 13*(2), 14-27.

Brennan, P., Moore, S., & Smyth, K. (1995). The effects of a special computer network on caregivers of persons with Alzheimer's disease. *Nursing Research, 44*(3), 166-172.

Finkler, S. (1992). *Budgeting concepts for nurse managers* (2nd ed.). Philadelphia: W. B. Saunders.

Finkler, S., & Kovner, C. (1993). *Financial management for nurse managers and executives.* Philadelphia: W. B. Saunders.

Garber, A. (1994). Can technology assessment control health spending? *Health Affairs, 13*(3), 115-126.

Gilbaldi, M., & Sullivan, S. (1994). A look at cost-effectiveness. *Pharmacotherapy, 14*(4), 399-414.

Hannah, K. (1988). Cost effectiveness analysis. In M. Ball, K. Hannah, U. Jelger, & H. Peterson (Eds.), *Informatics: Where caring and technology meet* (p. 225). New York: Springer.

Levin, H. (1983). *Cost effectiveness: A primer.* Beverly Hills, CA: Sage.

McGuire, R. C. (1995). *Cost effectiveness analysis of computer technology used in support of caregivers of patients with Alzheimer's disease.* Unpublished master's thesis, University of Kentucky, Lexington.

Mindel, C., Wright, R., & Starrett, R. (1986). Informal and formal health and social support systems of black and white elderly: A comparative cost approach. *The Gerontologist, 26*(3), 279-285.

Neumann, P., & Johannesson, M. (1994). From principle to public policy: Using cost-effectiveness analysis. *Health Affairs, 13*(3), 206-214.

U.S. Department of Commerce, Economics and Statistics Administration, Bureau of the Census. (1994). *Statistical Abstract of the United States 1994* (114th ed.). Washington, DC: Author.

U.S. Public Health Service. (1990). *Budget proposal; ComputerLink project* (PHS Form 398; Grant Number R01-AG08617-13). Washington, DC: Author.

CHAPTER 13

Maximizing Clinical Management Nationally Through Automation of the Federal Minimum Data Set

Christine M. Kowalski

The concept of a national Minimum Data Set moved into the long-term care industry as of 1990 with the inception of the Minimum Data Set (MDS) designed through the Health Care Finance Administration (HCFA). HCFA and the MDS design team planned for automation of the data and utilization of the information to manage the industry. The implementation evolution has gathered more than 3 years of concrete assessment information from all long-term care nursing homes/centers across the nation enrolled in a Medicare or Medicaid program. For the majority of persons collecting the MDS data, utilizing the data has been challenging because of the lack of automation and the minimal resources to compile the data into a useful format. Despite the challenges in using the data, changing health care forums such as subacute centers, the advancing levels of patient acuity, and managed care agencies requesting similar outcome measurements of shorter stay extended care residents, the need to utilize the centralized information is rapidly approaching. The need to evaluate quality of care, determine efficiency with quality unchanged, and advancement of nursing practice through outcome analysis is also driving long-term care companies, federal and state agencies, and independent organizations to collect patient/resident data. The availability of the MDS information now makes research much more possible and easier. This chapter will explore the uses of the MDS information to benefit the management of nursing home facilities and corporations.

As of 1990, the "long-term care" arm of inpatient health care has had the benefit of collecting a national standard transdisciplinary assessment commonly referred to as the Minimum Data Set (MDS; see Appendix A). The data collected encompass more than 100 items with over 400 possible responses to the items. The MDS content includes reviews of typical social service background and lifestyle questions, activity style, eating patterns, cognitive level, behaviors demonstrated, clinical care needs (basic activity of daily living needs), rehabilitation needs, skin care, and many functional assessment areas. The data are collected during the first 14 days of admission, quarterly, with any significant changes (as defined by HCFA), and annually. A 14-day assessment period allows sufficient time for evaluation of the person in various situations and also allows for adjustment to the new living arrangement.

The ultimate goal is for all nursing centers (also known as nursing homes or extended care facilities or locations providing care under a skilled nursing facility certificate/licensure, typically to the elderly population) to collect the data using an automated system and to submit the data through electronic transfer to the Health Care Finance Administration. Many corporations providing care through ownership of a large number of nursing centers set out to be automated as of October 1993. The requirement for manual completion of the standardized Minimum Data Set has been in place for more than 3 years in the long-term care arena. Automation requirements of the MDS are in place in several states (e.g., Pennsylvania, Washington, Texas, Indiana, and Ohio) across the United States for the purpose of reimbursing nursing homes participating in the Medicaid program and preparing survey teams with statistical data. In addition, there was a national effort to have all state agencies collect MDS data electronically by mid-1997, followed by submission from the state agencies to HCFA by early 1998. A committee organized by HCFA with representation from state agencies, facility-based staff, and information system designers has been developing the data collection functional requirements and all data submission standards that will be required for MDS data to be fed to the national database.

The concept of the national Minimum Data Set has moved the long-term care industry forward in the information system environment. Similar to the Nursing Minimum Data Set (NMDS), which was built upon the concept of the Uniform Minimum Health Data Sets (UMHDSs), the MDS was formed with the intent of capturing the "minimum set of items, with uniform definitions and categories" (Werley & Lang, 1988). Unlike the NMDS or UMHDSs, the MDS does not consider clinical populations other than the elderly, and it focuses on those in a nursing home setting. The data elements do establish a foundation for comparability of nursing data, which already has stimulated nursing research, but the content does not fully capture the treatment plans for an individual and partially gathers the intensity of nursing care.

To the present, the use of the data has been evolving and has become a significant tool for clinical management. The MDS provides a mechanism for organizations to evaluate themselves against other providers, identify quality improvement areas, and allow a scientifically established financial reimbursement system. The design of the MDS allows the care needs of the elderly population to drive the funding scale. Several Medicaid agencies collect MDS data monthly or quarterly, and based upon the items identified in the MDS, a monthly or quarterly rate is established and will remain in place until the next submission of data is evaluated.

Within the elderly community the idea of "long-term care" (LTC) has changed. No longer is the "feeble" older person needing minimal care entering the traditional nursing centers. Centers now resemble the medical/surgical unit previously housed in a hospital. The impact of the shift in this population has created several challenges for the LTC industry. This evolution for the nursing centers now includes advanced rehabilitation, subacute care units, specialty areas for Alzheimer's care, and wound care, as well as diversified areas such as high-risk pregnancy and burn care. To accommodate these changes, the need for data has become as important in the extended care arena as it has in the acute care settings. Recognizing the need for a uniform data collection tool, the Health Care Finance Administration has formalized a mandatory transdisciplinary assessment—now known as the MDS—for use in the United States.

HISTORY

In the nursing home reform law of the Omnibus Budget Reconciliation Act of 1987 (OBRA 87), the intent was to provide an opportunity to ensure good clinical practice by creating a regulatory framework that recognizes the importance of a comprehensive resident assessment as the foundation for planning and delivering care to every resident (U.S. Department of Health and Human Services' RAI Manual, 1995). The intent of the mandatory uniform assessment tool, the Minimum Data Set, is to provide a sound, standardized form to evaluate the health care of the elderly throughout the United States. The important provision of OBRA 87 was that the developers must design a Resident Assessment Instrument (RAI) that will be completed periodically on a routine basis. The RAI consists of the MDS, Resident Assessment Protocols (RAPs), and a corresponding care plan to identify actual or potential care issues (Figure 13.1) (Morris, Hawes, Fries, et al., 1991).

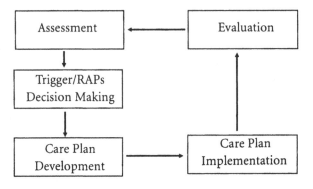

Figure 13.1. RAI Process

In MDS software and manually, answers from the MDS are mapped to a complex legend identifying "triggers" that ultimately note problem areas for the person assessed. Based upon the combinations of answers given, a list of potential problematic areas could be identified and categorized into a model titled Resident Assessment Protocols (RAPs). Once triggered, areas requiring further clinical evaluation (through an interdisciplinary team approach) would determine the need for a care plan.

A well-established team of experts on aging was granted the responsibility of developing the methodology design for the assessment tool and elderly care requirements. Embedded in the design of the form and the process was a goal to require related automation. Once each center had the automation, each state agency would gather the MDS information and then proceed to forward appropriate data to the federal government agency.

The MDS project has included a paper version of the tool with implementation across the country in *every* nursing home certified for Medicare and/or Medicaid reimbursement. Various states and research projects added to or changed the original form, resulting in multiple variations. To compensate for this, HCFA developed the MDS 2.0 version (discussed below) and prevented states from changing the core content of the form. Extensions of the original MDS project have brought drafts of the form to arenas including home health care, short stay clients, and international health care areas.

Expanding the first portion of the MDS project, information gathered through the Resident Assessment Instrument (RAI) process has assisted researchers at the University of Wisconsin-Madison, Center for Health Systems

Research and Analysis (CHSRA) in the development and implementation of a "case-mix" classification system, which has served as a basis for Medicaid and Medicare reimbursement. These researchers have also been working on a universal mechanism for using the information to assist with the nursing home survey process known as Quality Indicators.

As of January 1996, a second version of the original MDS, called MDS 2.0, was developed. All states have been required to convert to the new form, with the exception of the states that have previously established electronic transmission of MDS data and financial reimbursement based upon the MDS. Use by *all* states is expected by 1998. The main difference in the new form is primarily content. An addition of a discharge and reentry reason for assessment has been included specifically for electronic submission clarification and tracking. Items have been added, changed, moved, and reconfigured in an effort to clarify clinical definitions, facilitate clinical continuity, and ensure compatibility with the data entry functions of computerization (Richards & Fitzgerald, 1996).

Multiple MDS formats have created the need to adapt software frequently. Software vendors or designers have had to maintain several separate yet similar automated data collection tools. As states meet the challenge of using the MDS 2.0 form by mid-1997, it can be projected that states will be retrieving data from all nursing centers at the end of 1998.

MOVING THE MDS
ASSESSMENT INTO MANAGEMENT

The best approach to advancing the MDS within the nursing center is to find useful and beneficial purposes for all persons involved. Practitioners must be able to measure and assess the effectiveness of what they do, as well as have a degree of ownership and control of the information they collect to improve the quality of patient care (Casey, 1994). Professionals must feel they are part of the process to improve the care based upon the data they are recording.

Because the MDS is comprehensive, complicated, has a lengthy design, and contains the requirement to utilize multiple specialized professionals to accomplish the transdisciplinary approach, the need to identify quality advantages from the MDS tool was imperative. As more labor was invested for completion of the form and related documentation, a decrease in direct patient care became a realistic possibility. Managers of facilities and corporations began asking what they could gain from this massive effort.

In an attempt to maximize the MDS's content, and as a result of the publication of work on Quality Indicators from the University of Wisconsin (CHSRA) group, the initial focus for many organizations was quality improvement. In many health care arenas, the lack of access to information has created a major hurdle impeding the important progress toward quality improvement. Casey (1993) remarks that the access to information is required to support the quality assessment and improvement process. To complement this, the Joint Commission on Accreditation of Healthcare Organizations (JCAHO) reveals that data held in a comparative database have the potential to play an important role in terms of benchmarking as a quality improvement strategy (JCAHO, 1993). From a management perspective, having an automated source of MDS data available provided management with the ability to move to the next step, that of showing people how to use the information. To advance corporations with strong quality improvement philosophies, establishing a goal to formulate a desire and a process for utilization of MDS data was a progressive step. Similarly, state and federal agencies were working on methods for evaluating the quality of nursing centers using MDS data. To be informed providers, therefore, nursing centers would need to capture the same data the survey agencies would collect.

Standard reports designed to identify key issues (e.g., infections, in-house pressure ulcers, dehydration, deterioration of cognition) guide managers on what needs immediate attention. Once an area is noted on paper, managers' responsibility for verifying the issue, planning the mechanism for changing the issue, and monitoring the improvement would be clear. Overlooking or avoiding areas needing improvement would be more difficult. The practice of identifying issues, setting an attainable goal, putting an action plan into place, and evaluating success mirrors the nursing process and is the practice recommended by the developers of the RAI process and survey teams evaluating the nursing centers. Because of MDS data availability and, as noted by Zimmerman and colleagues (1995), by providing better information to the nursing home survey process, the survey teams can use key data collected off-site to prepare in identifying areas of potential concern or can utilize the processes on-site when reviewing facility records and quality of resident care warranting special focus. If nursing centers use the MDS data simultaneously, they can improve internal areas of concern and reduce the need for survey evaluation.

CORPORATE EVALUATION OF DATA:
CASE STUDY

In a corporation spreading across more than 10 states in the United States and divided into three districts, management staff initially used 66 items to track center quality improvement or potential areas of decline. Nursing consultants overseeing area operations would review the 66 items and focus on 10 or 12 key elements with the direct managers in the nursing center. As the acuity of residents changed and the repeated usage of "key" areas became the focal points of resident care, correlations between care and outcomes were noted more clearly. To assist in correlating data, the corporate clinical staff determined the need for up-to-date centralized data, in a manageable quantity and following the focal points of the nurse consultants. Likewise, reimbursement stakeholders were interested in the data as a matter of how the clients were improving and over what duration of time. As more data were collected, trends for caring for persons with different diagnoses or at different levels of care could be identified, as well as potential cost saving areas.

The most utilized reports were those identifying the key indicators. Items such as the number of residents physically or chemically restrained within the building, the number of pressure ulcers developing in the center, number of falls, usage of antipsychotic medications, and infection rate could be noted clearly on this report. These key items were tracked weekly in the subacute centers and monthly in the skilled nursing facilities. To assist in key area problem resolution, specialty reports could be produced easily to assist in determining the use of particular activity sessions, resident likes and dislikes of events, an activity of daily living (ADL) decline, potential social and psychiatric tendencies, and discharge needs, as well as others.

Nurses overseeing the districts and supervisors to the nurse consultants were charged with reviewing the content and assisting the nurse consultants and centers with problem solving and with prioritizing key areas for improvement. Quality Improvement Specialists, based out of the corporate office, reviewed the data prior to site visits to note areas needing critical review and reinforcement by the area or district supervisors. Upper management reviewed the content to compare regions, districts, and the corporation for trends of improvement and of decline. Clinical Advancement Teams utilized the data to determine areas of concentration for program development and product enhancement. Executives reviewed the data to compare the company with other providers and to determine new areas for expansion.

QUALITY INDICATOR DEVELOPMENT

As the MDS demonstration project data collection progressed, the data were to be utilized for the development of scientific quality indicators. Potential problematic "markers" of clinical practice were identified using data extracted from the MDS Plus design (an alternative form). The quality indicator development resulted from the growing interest of health care professionals, consumers, policymakers, and advocates in measuring the quality of care and quality of life of nursing home residents. The indicators were developed through a systematic approach involving extensive interdisciplinary clinical input, empirical analysis, and field testing. This approach resulted in 12 Care "Domains" and quality indicators considered "risk areas." The risk areas are adjusted for the expectedness and unexpectedness of a person falling into these areas, based on scientific calculations using specific selections contained within the MDS form (Zimmerman et al., 1995).

The domains cover 12 areas:

- Accidents
- Behavioral and emotional patterns
- Clinical management
- Cognitive patterns
- Elimination and continence
- Infection control
- Nutrition and eating
- Physical functioning
- Psychotropic drug use
- Quality of life
- Sensory function and communication
- Skin care

Areas such as Elimination and Continence were designed to assist the centers in determining the prevalence of bowel and bladder incontinence. Once the MDS results are gathered, data may be utilized to develop national statistics and allow individual centers to benchmark themselves against the nation. Falling within the domains are the 30 Quality Indicators that will become a national standardized measurement for nursing homes across the United States (Appendix B).

QUALITY INDICATOR USAGE:
CASE STUDY

Once the domains and risk factors were identified, it was evident that a new methodology for the state survey process was inevitable. As design for the MDS 2.0 software began, anticipation of the quality indicators was considered. Rather than developing a straightforward list, the goal was to encourage the field to "compile" the data with a management perspective. Previous reports identified the numbers of each element requested. New reports were designed through teams of staff representing various levels of management and different geographic areas, and who best understood the comprehensive process of the MDS 2.0 and its features. Elements were no longer looked at individually. The focus was to show how elements related to one another and to identify potential correlations of data. For example: Was incontinence related to a repetitive urinary tract infection or was it a physiological problem?

Reports using the content in a comparison format took on a matrix design. Easy identification of trends could be noted with multiple "X" marks under the same individual's name or the same nursing unit. Program and education series could be directed toward the trends noted within the matrices (Table 13.1).

As quality indicators became finalized, similar types of matrices were developed using the domains established by Zimmerman et al. (1995). The automation took into consideration the manually developed equations needed for identifying the risk factors of several indicators, thus removing the responsibility from the end user for calculating the risk potential.

In day-to-day practice, identification of the quality indicators and corporate indicators were utilized as issue identifiers and improvement notification. As designed, routine practice of the facility manager shared a prioritized list of potential issues, followed the nursing process, and, upon solution identification, allowed the center to share the results. With corrected practices in place, similar issues could be prevented from happening in the future, thus improving the overall function of the nursing center.

Monthly quality assurance and improvement meetings with key staff, including the medical director of the building, reviewed the data formally and compared data over time. Monthly, the manageable focus of one or two key areas would be identified with a mechanism for improving identified. All staff were made aware of the monthly goal. Approaches toward the goals were reasonable and realistic.

Management staff were charged with coaching the frontline staff when needed and with sharing success stories publicly. Newsletters often included the goals of the previous quarter and the results of the problem-solving approach. Likewise, corporate goals were established and district teams noted the goals in weekly update calls/visits with each center. Goals were set, and the standards for each goal were based upon a national or corporate average. An example of a corporate goal was to "achieve an average of zero for pressure ulcers within the corporation."

Using the MDS Quality Indicator Process (see Figure 13.2), preparation by the nursing center for the state annual survey became less labor intensive. Ongoing monitoring proved to be worthwhile for the survey process. Areas of concern noted often during a survey would have previously been recognized and an action plan(s) in place. With the continual observation of facility trends,

TABLE 13.1   Resident Weight/Nutrition Matrix

Resident Name	Room	Wght Loss/Gain	Previous Weight	Most Current Weight	Oral Problems	Diet Supplement	Tube Feeding	Assist w/ Eating
A. D.	400B	5+	190 (10/20)	195 (11/20)	X			X
B. J.	410B	10+ **	150 (9/24)	160 (10/22)	X	X	X	
F. B.	409A	5+	172 (10/01)	177 (11/13)		X		X
G. M.	418A	−5 **	135 (10/20)	130 (11/15)	X	X		X

NOTE: ** Indicates significant percentage of weight loss/gain within time boundaries.

key areas were not allowed to slip through the cracks. Sharing responsibility among staff members during the design and implementation of the action plans made all staff aware of the issues, assisted them in solving by providing recommendations for improvement, and allowed them to see successes through the positive reinforcement of information sharing.

ADDITIONAL MANAGEMENT USES
FOR THE MINIMUM DATA SET

In researching data from the MDS, developers and users found the data also identified levels of illness. Several groups were interested in identifying a person's level of cognitive deterioration or dementia. An MDS Cognitive Scale, MDS-COGS, was developed by a group of researchers. Similar work was done by the developers of the MDS in the design of the Cognitive Performance Scale. These scales have been incorporated into dementia programs across the nation. The MDS-COGS provides a valid measure of the presence and severity of a person's cognitive impairment based upon data contained within the MDS instrument. Although cognitive instruments are available in great number and are able to determine the severity level for dementia, they often are not practical for the LTC environment. The problem relates to the availability of highly skilled professionals to conduct the test, and to costs associated with this service.

A tool such as MDS-COGS benefits the industry by allowing the information from the MDS to be applied to a scale so a measure of severity can be determined. Research has shown the tool to be an effective measurement instrument able to replace the commonly known mini-mental exam utilized frequently in the nursing home industry.

For managers, the MDS-COGS provides a simple, direct, and easily available scale. Because the MDS information is mandatory, the information for the scale calculations is easily available and can be computed through an automated system. Because professionally trained staff are not required in order to obtain

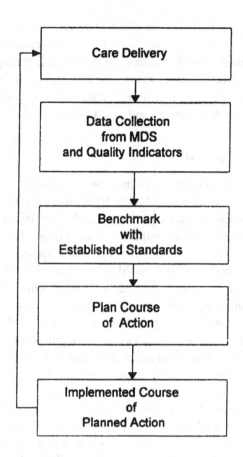

Figure 13.2. MDS Quality Indicator Process

this information, the administrative costs are minimal. Interpretation is straightforward and can be repeated with each assessment.

The scale identifies memory problems, orientation level, ability to make decisions, communication patterns, and physical functioning. Using a simple scale ranging from 1 to 10, the staff are quickly able to identify the level of care needed for a cognitively impaired person along with the appropriate placement in dementia programs (Hartmaier, Sloane, Guess, & Koch, 1994).

As the great need for research and trending relating to the area of incontinence in the LTC industry continued, the MDS content was looked at again. The MDS provided a group of researchers the ability to compare the MDS incontinence scoring to geographic areas, methods of care, and policies for incontinence (Crooks, Schnelle, Ouslander, & McNees, 1995). The centralized database for corporations will provide the ability to trial new programs in an area such as incontinence and to evaluate the effectiveness through random sample analysis in a region, a state, or under the direction of certain management. The MDS provides management with a sound base of information to analyze practice standards objectively and to test new methods.

PROCESS CONSIDERATIONS

As the MDS evolved and data usage increased, a deficit of data accuracy became evident. The process established by HCFA for completing the form required the form to be done at least quarterly, with the exception of significant change in conditions. Because corporations wanted to keep data more current and reflective of the residents, assessments were often updated between the required quarterly time frames and stored as a separate file. The workload addition was a concern to managers and staff around the country. To meet the required documentation minimum and to ease the documentation required for tracking purposes within a corporation, it was planned that the least amount of updating would be set in the automation process of the MDS. To accomplish both goals, a process was established to have weekly updates placed into the computer system on the "critical areas" that would feed the "key reports."

Complications developed when the criteria to keep each file distinct from others and the need to develop a process for "locking" the information arose. Once a file was "locked," no changes were allowed and printing was required. To accomplish the transdisciplinary approach for completing the MDS, multiple disciplines needed to have their required content completed prior to the 14-day cutoff. If the information was not completed on the computer, the person "finalizing" the form could not lock the file due to the "omissions." Because the completion date is set by HCFA and survey teams audit the data during their visits, strict adherence to the completion date of the file was required. Unfortunately, in a fast-paced, changing environment, the available computer time could not always be found and as a result the MDS form would appear with omissions and the finalization of the file could not occur in a timely manner. To assist with identifying the omissions, an automated "error reporting" system was designed by vendors. This "error reporting" allows the person "finalizing" the file to note both which items have been omitted and proof for any "impossible" combinations of data—such as a selection for comatose and another noting alert. If all the items are in place, the process takes seconds. If the items are not in place, the coordinator must gather a list of missing items from the clinical computer system, track down the person(s) responsible for the incomplete field(s), wait until they are able to complete the information, and then repeat the error-checking process. In a realistic environment, it is more likely that the latter process occurs and that the completion time is extended and made more complex.

Conceptually, the locking process was a great step toward ensuring data in a structured format; upon implementation, however, the process became cumbersome, complex, and often incorrectly done. Files were often not locked, and previous files were written over. Correct report generation became complex because the locked data were the "registered" information, yet, due to the need to update files in between required assessments, the last set of elements placed in the computer system became the most current information. Reports were designed to pull from the "registered/locked" information although the user knew the resident "picture" was different than the report. The difference in the results began to create disbelief in the data and to confuse the person(s) using the reports. To resolve the issues, each file was closed and locked within 5 days, even if incomplete.

INFORMATION SYSTEMS CONSIDERATIONS

Database development based on the form design created complexities. HCFA allowed system designers to structure the form presentation in any manner they desired. As a form, however, the output structure required that it be delivered in the mandated format. Initially, the content was incorporated into a "comprehensive assessment," which covered more than the items on the MDS form. As the "comprehensive assessment" was used more and more, concerns regarding the overwhelming amount of detail and the inability to navigate quickly through the computer system to access necessary material were expressed. Similarly, it was confusing for persons being trained on the MDS content to follow the computer screen because the screen did not follow the sequence of the manual HCFA form. To assist the user with these concerns, the software was rewritten to reflect the sequence of the MDS form, and the comprehensive content was placed in specific departmental assessments.

Designing software to meet the user-friendly requirements was challenging. Although the format was standardized and data specifications were supplied by HCFA, some state agencies moved the content into a different form layout or added new content that resulted in new pages to the original form. Programmers were responsible for maintaining a similar appearance and data entry mechanism for each state variation. Similarly, with automation as a long-range goal, design for maintaining a standardized database structure was a necessity.

Having the Clinical Services Department working with the Information Services Department was vital to the success of the design so that clinical interpretations of guidelines were incorporated into the information system and
consideration of the fast-paced environment was included.

The design of a "locking" mechanism was important to the system and yet
created complexities for the user. It was determined that because of having the
file secured by a completion date and the need to transmit files cleanly to the
state agencies, the process was not an option. The decision for file locking was
supported by HCFA in the automation functional requirements publication of
the MDS 2.0.

Electronic data transfer requirements continue to evolve as more states set
a goal for MDS transmission. Standardization of this transmission is being
planned at the federal level, but many states are trying to forge ahead and are
developing their own criteria. As a result, corporations and vendors will need
to support the multiple state variations. These variations not only create an
additional workload but also additional maintenance of the various systems,
which indirectly results in revenue losses.

For the global outcomes and quality indicator analysis of corporate data, the
retrieval and archiving of data required a submission process to the centralized
database. So that corporations can be competitive in the LTC market, a central
data warehouse has been identified as a necessity for conducting queries on
facility information and to establish benchmarks. To accomplish this centralized data warehouse, it was necessary to identify that each state has their own
electronic submission mechanisms and that the linkages to the corporate pool
would need to accommodate those variations. From the executive viewpoint,
the data will provide a great source of information for activity-based costing,
contract and program evaluation, and quality improvement research.

COST INFORMATION

Automation of the MDS was an expectation of long-term care providers. In
a survey conducted for *McKnight's Long Term Care News* (O'Connor, 1994) as
of June 1994, it was found that 65% of the nation's state association members
had implemented a computer system relating to their patient care functions.
The expected outlay of funds for automation per nursing center is approximately $25,000. For the industry, the projected cost is greater than $270 million
dollars for equipment and software to meet the regulations. Benefits of the
automation will assist HCFA's overseeing of facility quality, allow for research,
and provide consumer information. For the facility, more efficiency and reduction in labor costs will result (O'Connor, 1994). To assist in the funding of the

project, some state agencies have agreed to or have already provided capital reimbursement of approximately $2,000 worth of equipment for centers actively participating in the Medicaid program and for those able to meet the required Medicaid capital expense criteria.

Corporations are expanding automation of nursing centers to comply with the regulatory environments, and a few have taken on the responsibility of owning and developing their software. Large contracts from major corporations often stretch the abilities of a small or midsize vendor and result in the inability to meet customer or regulatory requirements in a timely fashion. Because of the difficulties in meeting deadlines and solving substantial software problems, corporations have brought the information service function "in-house." Smaller groups of facilities or stand-alone nursing centers generally do not have this luxury and are faced with using the software as it is delivered.

For corporations choosing to develop software internally, the cost for programming and maintenance of systems has expanded the information technology budgets significantly. Information system departments within the industry have now grown from between 3 and 5 employees to more than 80 employees in some larger corporations. Responsibilities extend from clinical to financial data management while encompassing software and hardware technical and support services.

CASE MIX REIMBURSEMENT

The Case Mix and Quality Demonstration Project was funded by HCFA for the purpose of developing and implementing a case-mix classification system that would serve as a basis for Medicaid and Medicare payment. The components of case mix reimbursement often consider inflation, property value and costs, clinical care needs (mostly nursing care, direct and indirect care), the cost center limits (maximum payment amounts), and occupancy percentage. These dollars are dispersed on a per diem basis considering the number of days residents are actually in the nursing facility per month or quarter (McDaniel, 1996).

The case mix classification system design is based on time studies and assessment information gathered from six states (Texas, Maine, Kansas, South Dakota, Mississippi, and New York). Originally, the classification entailed 44 areas and was known as the RUGs-III (Resource Utilization Groups) system. Each state developed a variation of the model and researched the pricing structure to accompany the clinical care identified. The result is based upon data submission from the MDS content and the reimbursement system. The outcome is a per diem payment rate (Collier, 1996). Using the MDS content and incorporating the administrative costs, a state will determine a daily dollar figure for each resident or an overall daily average for the entire nursing center. The data are electronically submitted to the state, and the number of days that the resident resided in the nursing facility are counted and multiplied by the daily rate. To obtain a rate for the center versus an individual, the daily rates for each resident are averaged. Once the reimbursement amount is established, it is sent to the provider on a monthly or quarterly basis (depending on the state process; see Table 13.2).

CASE MIX CLASSIFICATION IMPACT

Features of the case mix information include statewide standard classification of long-term care residents, annual cost reporting, annual rate structuring, an equitable payment system, improved management practices, improved quality of care, and clinical outcomes. For the management staff, the case mix classification system provided a clear picture of the cost of resident care in the nursing centers.

The answers provided in the MDS form gained a greater importance when the relationship to reimbursement became a reality. Managers initially had to scrutinize each form to ensure that the resident status was reflected accurately and that the person completing the form understood the content definitions as they were intended. Instruction of staff included several sessions identifying the key factors moving residents from each level of the classification system and reviewed the definitions to questions and answers on the MDS, thereby emphasizing the importance of conscientious assessments. Amendments to MDS data may or may not be allowed after review by the state collection center. If amendments are allowed, some states will allow only a percentage of items be incorrect before penalties are put into place. If a penalty is put into place, it could mean a substantial loss to the provider, and it is therefore avoided at all costs.

CONCLUSION

With the inception of the MDS and its related processes, the door has been opened to automation for the long-term care arena. The ability for clinical managers to capitalize on data that is collected in a routine, standard manner is now available. The problem of not having data available in an automated fashion is no longer a stumbling block for clinical research. The goals of monitoring nursing care and resident outcomes can more easily be the focus of a manager's role. With experience, collecting the data using a computer input

TABLE 13.2   Case Mix Reimbursement Rate Summary Example

Item 1	Direct care and care-related per diem	$34.56
Item 2	Administrative and operating per diem	$24.29
Item 3	Property cost per diem	$6.68
Item 4	Return on equity capital per diem	$0.89
Total (per resident) Rate:	Jan. 1-Mar. 31, 1996	$66.42

device will become second nature to the field staff. Progress will be made in advancing clinical software to calculate and organize the wealth of information and ultimately improve nursing practice.

The industry continues to measure success by achieving paper compliance. The next step is to have clinical managers think "out of the box." To advance the facility practice, an internal paradigm shift will need to occur whereby the staff will understand the benefits of completing an MDS form and utilizing the RAI process to truly improve a resident's quality of care and quality of life. Once quality of care and quality of life are recognized, the new internal "systems" will need to be ingrained with the ongoing care. The MDS is a tool that has moved the long-term care industry ahead in terms of uniform data collection and has set a standard for how automation and an electronic data bank can be established. It is now the industry's responsibility to utilize the data to its fullest and advance the practice accordingly.

Appendix A
Minimum Data Set

Resident _____ Numeric Identifier _____

MINIMUM DATA SET (MDS) —*VERSION 2.0*
FOR NURSING HOME RESIDENT ASSESSMENT AND CARE SCREENING
FULL ASSESSMENT FORM
(Status in last 7 days, unless other time frame indicated)

SECTION A. IDENTIFICATION AND BACKGROUND INFORMATION

1. **RESIDENT NAME** — a. (First) b. (Middle Initial) c. (Last) d. (Jr/Sr)

2. **ROOM NUMBER**

3. **ASSESSMENT REFERENCE DATE** — a. *Last day of MDS observation period* Month Day Year
   b. Original (0) or corrected copy of form (enter number of correction)

4a. **DATE OF REENTRY** — Date of reentry from most recent temporary discharge to a hospital in last 90 days (or since last assessment or admission if less than 90 days) Month Day Year

5. **MARITAL STATUS** — 1. Never married 2. Married 3. Widowed 4. Separated 5. Divorced

6. **MEDICAL RECORD NO.**

7. **CURRENT PAYMENT SOURCES FOR N.H. STAY** — *(Billing Office to indicate; check all that apply in last 30 days)*
   Medicaid per diem   a.
   Medicare per diem   b.
   Medicare ancillary part A   c.
   Medicare ancillary part B   d.
   CHAMPUS per diem   e.
   VA per diem   f.
   Self or family pays for full per diem   g.
   Medicaid resident liability or Medicare co-payment   h.
   Private insurance per diem (including co-payment)   i.
   Other per diem   j.

8. **REASONS FOR ASSESSMENT** *[Note - If this is a discharge or reentry assessment, only a limited subset of MDS items need be completed]*
   a. Primary reason for assessment
   1. Admission assessment (required by day 14)
   2. Annual assessment
   3. Significant change in status assessment
   4. Significant correction of prior full assessment
   5. Quarterly review assessment
   10. Significant correction of prior quarterly assessment
   6. Discharged--return not anticipated
   7. Discharged--return anticipated
   8. Discharged prior to completing initial assessment
   9. Reentry
   0. NONE OF ABOVE
   b. Special codes for use with supplemental assessment types in Case Mix demonstration states or other states where required
   1. 5 day assessment
   2. 30 day assessment
   3. 60 day assessment
   4. Quarterly assessment using full MDS form
   5. Readmission/return assessment
   6. Other state required assessment

9. **RESPONSIBILITY/ LEGAL GUARDIAN** — *(Check all that apply)*
   Legal Guardian   a.
   Other legal oversight   b.
   Durable power of attorney/health care   c.
   Durable power attorney/financial   d.
   Family member responsible   e.
   Patient responsible for self   f.
   NONE OF ABOVE   g.

10. **ADVANCED DIRECTIVES** *(For those items with supporting documentation in the medical record, check all that apply)*
    Living will   a.
    Do not resuscitate   b.
    Do not hospitalize   c.
    Organ donation   d.
    Autopsy request   e.
    Feeding restrictions   f.
    Medication restrictions   g.
    Other treatment restrictions   h.
    NONE OF THE ABOVE   i.

SECTION B. COGNITIVE PATTERNS

1. **COMATOSE** *(Persistent vegetative state/no discernible consciousness)*
   0. No   1. Yes   (If yes, skip to Section G)

2. **MEMORY** *(Recall of what was learned or known)*
   a. Short-term memory OK--seems/appears to recall after 5 minutes
   0. Memory OK   1. Memory problem
   b. Long-term memory OK--seems/appears to recall long past
   0. Memory OK   1. Memory problem

3. **MEMORY/ RECALL ABILITY** — *Check all that resident was normally able to recall during last 7 days)*
   Current season   a.
   Location of own room   b.
   Staff names/faces   c.
   That he/she is in a nursing home   d.
   None of the Above are recalled   e.

4. **COGNITIVE SKILLS FOR DAILY DECISION-MAKING** *(Made decisions regarding tasks of daily life)*
   0. INDEPENDENT--decisions consistent/reasonable
   1. MODIFIED INDEPENDENCE--some difficulty in new situations only
   2. MODERATELY IMPAIRED--decisions poor; cues/supervision required
   3. SEVERELY IMPAIRED--never/rarely made decisions

5. **INDICATORS OF DELIRIUM-- PERIODIC DISORDERED THINKING/ AWARENESS** *(Code for behavior in the last 7 days.) (Note: Accurate assessment requires conversations with staff and family who have direct knowledge of resident's behavior over this time).*
   0. Behavior not present
   1. Behavior present, not of recent onset
   2. Behavior present, over last 7 days appears different from resident's usual functioning (e.g., new onset or worsening)
   a. EASILY DISTRACTED--(e.g. difficulty paying attention; gets sidetracked)
   b. PERIODS OF ALTERED PERCEPTION OR AWARENESS OF SURROUNDINGS--(e.g., moves lips or talks to someone not present; believes he/she is somewhere else; confuses night and day)
   c. EPISODES OF DISORGANIZED SPEECH--(e.g., speech is incoherent, nonsensical, irrelevant, or rambling from subject to subject; loses train of thought)
   d. PERIODS OF RESTLESSNESS--(e.g., fidgeting or picking at skin, clothing, napkins, etc.; frequent position changes; repetitive physical movements or calling out)
   e. PERIODS OF LETHARGY--(e.g., sluggishness; staring into space; difficult to arouse; little body movement)
   f. MENTAL FUNCTION VARIES OVER THE COURSE OF THE DAY--(e.g., sometimes better; sometimes worse; behaviors sometimes present, sometimes not)

6. **CHANGE IN COGNITIVE STATUS** — Resident's cognitive status, skills, or abilities have changed as compared to status of 90 days ago (or since last assessment if less than 90 days)
   0. No change   1. Improved   2. Deteriorated

SECTION C. COMMUNICATION/HEARING PATTERNS

1. **HEARING** *(With hearing appliance, if used)*
   0. HEARS ADEQUATELY--normal talk, TV, phone
   1. MINIMAL DIFFICULTY when not in quiet setting
   2. HEARS IN SPECIAL SITUATIONS ONLY--speaker has to adjust tonal quality and speak distinctly
   3. HIGHLY IMPAIRED/absence of useful hearing

2. **COMMUNICATION DEVICES/ TECHNIQUES** *(Check all that apply during last 7 days)*
   Hearing aid, present and used   a.
   Hearing aid, present but not used regularly   b.
   Other receptive comm. techniques used (e.g., lip reading)   c.
   NONE OF THE ABOVE   d.

3. **MODES OF EXPRESSION** *(Check all used by resident to make needs known)*
   Speech   a.
   Writing messages to express or clarify needs   b.
   American sign language or Braille   c.
   Signs/gestures/sounds   d.
   Communication board   e.
   Other   f.
   NONE OF THE ABOVE   g.

4. **MAKING SELF UNDERSTOOD** *(Expressing information content--however able)*
   0. UNDERSTOOD
   1. USUALLY UNDERSTOOD-- difficulty finding words or finishing thoughts
   2. SOMETIMES UNDERSTOOD--ability is limited to making concrete requests
   3. RARELY/NEVER UNDERSTOOD

5. **SPEECH CLARITY** *(Code for speech in the last 7 days)*
   0. CLEAR SPEECH--distinct, intelligible words
   1. UNCLEAR SPEECH--slurred, mumbled words
   2. NO SPEECH--absence of spoken words

6. **ABILITY TO UNDERSTAND OTHERS** *(Understanding verbal information content--however able)*
   0. UNDERSTANDS
   1. USUALLY UNDERSTANDS--may miss some part/intent of message
   2. SOMETIMES UNDERSTANDS--responds adequately to simple, direct communication
   3. RARELY/NEVER UNDERSTANDS

7. **CHANGE IN COMMUNICATION/ HEARING** — Resident's ability to express, understand, or hear information has changed as compared to status of 90 days ago (or since last assessment if less than 90 days)
   0. No change   1. Improved   2. Deteriorated

☐ = When box blank, must enter number or letter   [a.] = When letter in box, check if condition applies   MDS 2.0 10/18/94

Appendix B
Quality Indicators and Risk Adjustment Used in Demonstration Facility

Domain	Quality Indicator	Type of Indicator	Risk Adjustment
Accidents	Prevalence of any injury	Outcome	No
	Prevalence of falls	Outcome	No
Behavioral and Emotional Patterns	Prevalence of problem behavior toward others	Outcome	Yes
	Prevalence of symptoms of depression	Outcome	No
	Prevalence of symptoms of depression with no treatment	Both	No
Clinical Management	Use of 9 or more scheduled medications	Process	No
Cognitive Patterns	Incidence of cognitive impairment	Outcome	No
Elimination and Continence	Prevalence of bladder or bowel incontinence	Outcome	Yes
	Prevalence of occasional bladder or bowel incontinence without a toileting plan	Both	No
	Prevalence of indwelling catheters	Process	Yes
	Prevalence of fecal impaction	Outcome	No
Infection Control	Prevalence of urinary tract infections	Outcome	No
	Prevalence of antibiotic or anti-infective use	Process	No
Nutrition and Eating	Prevalence of weight loss	Outcome	No
	Prevalence of tube feeding	Process	No
	Prevalence of dehydration	Outcome	No
Physical Functioning	Prevalence of bedfast residents	Outcome	No
	Incidence of decline in late-loss activities of daily living	Outcome	Yes
	Incidence of contractures	Outcome	Yes
	Lack of training or skill practice or range of motion for mobility-dependent residents	Both	No
Psychotropic Drug Use	Prevalence of antipsychotic use in the absence of psychotic and related conditions	Process	Yes
	Prevalence of antipsychotic daily dose in excess of surveyor guidelines	Process	No
	Prevalence of antianxiety or hypnotic drug use	Process	No
	Prevalence of hypnotic drug use on a scheduled or as-needed basis greater than twice in last week	Process	No
	Prevalence of use of any long-acting benzodiazepine	Process	No
Quality of Life	Prevalence of daily physical restraints	Process	No
	Prevalence of little or no activity	Outcome	No
Sensory Function and Communication	Lack of corrective action for sensory or communications problems	Both	No
Skin Care	Prevalence of stage 1-4 pressure ulcers	Outcome	Yes
	Insulin-dependent diabetes with no foot care	Both	No

SOURCE: Zimmerman et al., Center for Health Systems Research and Analysis, University of Wisconsin-Madison, 1995
NOTE: Late-loss activities of daily living are bed mobility, eating, toileting, and transfer.

REFERENCES

Casey, A. (1994). The UK clinical terms projects and quality improvement. In S. B. Henry, W. L. Holzemer, M. Tallberg, & S. J. Grobe (Eds.), *Informatics: The infrastructure for quality assessment and improvement in nursing* (p. 21). San Francisco: UC Nursing Press.

Collier, J. (1996). From assessment claims: How to set up a case mix payment system in your state. In *Case mix: A strong foundation for quality care* (pp. 37-40). Dallas: Texas Department of Human Services.

Crooks, V. C., Schnelle, J. F., Ouslander, J. P., & McNees, M. P. (1995). Use of the Minimum Data Set to rate incontinence severity. *Journal of the American Geriatrics Society, 43*(12), 1363-1369.

Hartmaier, S. L., Sloane, P. D., Guess, H. A., & Koch, G. G. (1994). The MDS Cognition Scale: A valid instrument for identifying and staging nursing home residents with dementia using the Minimum Data Set. *Journal of the American Geriatric Society, 42*(11), 1173-1179.

Joint Commission on Accreditation of Healthcare Organizations. (1993). *1994 manual: Accreditation manual for hospitals.* Chicago: Author.

McDaniel, B. (1996). From assessment claims: How to set up a case mix payment system in your state. In *Case mix: A strong foundation for quality care* (pp. 6-17). Dallas: Texas Department of Human Services.

Morris, J. N., Hawes, C., Fries, B. E., et al. (1991). *Resident assessment instrument training manual and resource guide.* Natick, MA: Eliot.

O'Connor, J. (1994). MDS automation mandate requires computerization. *McKnight's Long Term Care News, 15*(6), 1, 4.

Richards, M. B., & Fitzgerald, P. (1996). Providers' perspective: The next generation of resident assessment. *Nursing Home Medicine, 4*(3), 93-96.

U.S. Department of Health and Human Services, Health Care Finance Administration. (1995). *Long term care resident assessment instrument user's manual* (pp. 1-2). Baltimore, MD: Author.

Werley, H., & Lang, N. (1988). *Identification of the Nursing Minimum Data Set.* New York: Springer.

Zimmerman, D. R., Karon, S. L., Arling, G., Ryther-Clark, B., Collins, T., Ross, R., & Sainfort, F. (1995). Developing and testing of nursing home quality indicators. *Health Care Financing Review, 16*(4), 107-113.

CHAPTER 14

Use of Nursing Information Systems in Community Settings

Gary Bargstadt

Information systems have been used in community settings since the beginning of modern nursing. They have tremendous capability for increasing an agency's effectiveness in providing service to individual clients, population groups, and communities. Information systems help agencies to organize data, evaluate the outcomes of services provided, compare and contrast the effectiveness of different approaches to service delivery, and standardize practice.

There are challenges to the use of data in information systems. These challenges include lack of a common nomenclature for staff in community settings to communicate clearly with each other. Lack of common definitions is a barrier to comparison of data between agencies. In addition, maintaining confidentiality of data becomes increasingly challenging as information from a common database is shared among agencies. Finally, the variety of software platforms available to users today can present challenges in sharing common data files.

OVERVIEW

Since the emergence of modern nursing, data about persons, groups, and communities have been collected. Florence Nightingale, founder of modern nursing, was a strong proponent of systematic observation and recording of both individual and community information. Her interest followed the work of William Rathbone in England in 1859. The outstanding care provided to his dying wife prompted Rathbone to conclude that people with long-term illnesses could best be cared for at home. His writings on this subject spurred Florence Nightingale to publish *Suggestions for Improving Nursing Service* (Stanhope & Lancaster, 1992, p. 7).

Early in the 20th century in the United States, Lillian Wald and Mary Brewster trained nurses and wealthy women to provide nursing service to the poor of New York. In addition, Lillian Wald established the first community health nursing program for workers at the Metropolitan Life Insurance Company. She convinced companies it would cost less to use the services of organized community health nurses than to employ their own (Stanhope & Lancaster, 1992, p. 8). Today, nurses have been interested in demonstrating that the application of concepts and propositions of nursing make a difference in the outcomes of nursing care for persons, groups, and communities. Hence, the quest for useful data in community health settings has been and continues to be significant to community health practitioners and administrators.

Information is the critical variable in the justification of the need for funding, the demonstration of the effects of nursing service, and the preparation of reports for the community. With advancing computer technology, nursing skills needed to collect and analyze data to produce community health information have improved. Initially, nurses used hand-tabulated statistical reports; they then advanced to the punched B-sort cards so popular for early computers. Today, sophisticated computer technology is available. Current technology assists nurses to justify the need for funding, to demonstrate outcomes of nursing care, and to aid in the preparation of community reports.

In the community setting, information systems capture data from three perspectives: (a) individual clients, (b) groups of clients, and (c) the community as client. The information needed to provide service to each group is similar, yet each has distinct differences. Information systems in community health must address data and issues for both the financial and the clinical needs arising from service to individuals, groups, and communities.

MANAGEMENT OF INDIVIDUAL CLIENT DATA

Individual client data are critical for providing safe and cost-effective care to each client. Individual client data are derived from a variety of sources. Information systems assist the practitioner in organizing data from multiple sources and facilitating communication among multiple users of that data.

In the community setting, assessment data are gathered about a client on admission and throughout the client's length of stay on agency service. These data are used to formulate an accurate picture of the client's health and social problems for the purpose of establishing a plan of care that will meet the client's needs. At the Visiting Nurse Service of Des Moines (VNS), information systems help the practitioner to organize information collected about a client into a meaningful format. The information system, Home Health DataPLUS, also transports collected data to the appropriate agency form, eliminating the need for the practitioner to make multiple entries of the same data. For example, upon admission to service at VNS, a client's vital signs are incorporated into the initial client assessment, reported back to the physician, documented in the initial clinical note of the nurse, and included in reports back to the third-party payer and the referral source. Rather than the practitioner documenting those vital signs in five places, the information system is capable of transporting these data to the appropriate places in the clinical documentation system with a single entry. In addition, the system produces reports that assist in measuring client outcomes, such as a change in the client's health status from admission to discharge.

A second use of information systems in providing care to individual clients is in organizing material to guide practice. In the past several years there has been a proliferation of clinical tools for staff in community settings. Disease management programs guide the practitioner in "best practices" for delivery of care to a client. These diagnostic-specific tools have been developed for major diagnoses of clients visited in a community setting. Incorporated into these tools are critical pathways of care for a client. Critical pathways provide a map or guide for the practitioner in delivery of care to clients. At VNS, the critical pathway provides information about the number of visits needed by each discipline for the "average" client to learn independent self-care. Parameters for data gathering on the initial and subsequent visits, patient teaching materials, and key measures for defining outcomes of client care are also a component of the clinical pathway.

Information systems have the capability of storing information related to specific disease processes and of assisting the practitioner in generating a client-specific plan of care with input from the client and members of other disciplines who provide care. When a client is admitted for service, the computer generates a suggested plan of care for the client's primary diagnosis. The plan of care is modified by the practitioner based upon that individual client's needs, other client diagnoses, and the client's internal and external resources.

Identification and accumulation of resource materials for staff to use in providing care is the third organizational use of information systems in providing care to individual clients. An important function of staff in a community setting is client education. Information systems have the potential of storing information that staff will use in client education and of having this information at the practitioner's disposal. There is a wealth of teaching materials related to disease processes, medications, treatments, and procedures. The information system at VNS has the capability of producing client teaching documents for the practitioner that are appropriate to the client's diagnoses, medication regime, and interdisciplinary care plan, including the physician's treatment plan.

COMMUNICATION

Information systems also facilitate communication among providers of care to clients. Frequently in a community setting more than one nurse will be providing care to an individual client or family. To provide safe, effective care to clients, it is imperative that client information be communicated to other nurses who are providing care to that client. An information system facilitates sharing of information among nurses. At VNS, the computer generates a plan of care with past visit information, including key indicators of the client's health status from the four previous visits. These key indicators include such information as the client's latest blood pressure readings or the last several wound measurements and descriptions. The computer generates a succinct summary of the client's current treatment and teaching plan as well as key information from the client's past visits. These summaries save the nurse time in communicating about client care while ensuring transfer of key information to those involved in the client's care.

In addition to sharing client information among nurses, it is imperative that information be shared with members of other disciplines involved in the client's care. Information systems permit easy flow of information among disciplines. For example, a nurse makes a referral for physical therapy. The data needed for the physical therapist to make the client visit are compiled by the computer system and printed or sent electronically to the therapist. This includes demographic information about the client, the nurse's assessment and plan of care, and key information from the initial or past nursing visits to the client. Once the therapist has completed a visit and initiated a plan of care, that information is keyed into the computer for access by other disciplines involved in the client's care.

Tracking individual client information is also critical for billing functions. In a managed care environment, the number of client visits is frequently authorized by a payer's case management staff in advance of providing care. A limited number of visits is typically authorized. Additional visits need prior approval of the funding source case manager. Although it is difficult to track large numbers of preauthorized visits for several clients manually, the computer provides a mechanism for tracking. Agency staff are notified when the authorization has expired or the number of preauthorized visits has been exhausted. The VNS computer system, Home Health DataPLUS, also performs a technical review of key funding source variables and agency documentation standards, identifying individual client records that need additional review or oversight. For example, at VNS, the computer completes a check of 117 items on each individual record prior to billing for service. A list is then generated of client records that have not passed this technical review. The list includes information about specific technical elements that are missing or incorrect. These are reviewed by the practitioner or manager and corrected prior to billing.

Finally, information systems can enhance communication for agency performance improvement activities and risk management. For example, it is prudent for agencies to monitor instances in which a client returns to the hospital within 30 days of discharge to home care. A listing of all clients who have been readmitted to a hospital within time parameters specified by the agency are reviewed by agency performance improvement staff, risk management staff, or both. Information gleaned from this review is helpful in determining if risk management issues are present for a specific client. Client outcomes also can be monitored for parameters specified by the agency. For example, a more in-depth review of individual client care plans and client progress is provided for clients who are on service longer than expected or for whom visit frequency is greater than anticipated.

Client information systems can enhance care to individual clients by organizing data obtained from multiple sources. These data can be organized in ways that make the practitioner's job easier and more rewarding. For example, information gathered from family members, physicians, case workers, and other health care providers regarding a client's care can be grouped together in a client database. This eliminates the problem of reading through several pages of text to find pertinent information.

There are also inherent problems in information systems as used with individual clients. Two such problems are

- lack of a common nomenclature for use among nurses and between disciplines
- a historical financial/statistical, as opposed to clinical, orientation of computer programs

A pressing problem encountered in communication of data among health care professionals is the lack of one accepted nomenclature for client problems in community health. Among classifications recognized by the American Nurses Association are North American Nursing Diagnosis Association (NANDA) and the Omaha System. Lack of a single common accepted nursing nomenclature makes it more difficult for staff to communicate about client problems. If staff at an acute care setting use NANDA and refer the client to a home care agency that uses the Omaha System, a question as to which nomenclature will be used to communicate information about the client between agencies emerges. Would the nurse use both systems? Some believe the NANDA nomenclature is better adapted for an acute care institutional setting than the Omaha System. Others believe the Omaha System's nomenclature is better suited for a community health environment because it addresses issues related to the persons' environment as well as their physiological, psychological, and behavioral status (Martin & Scheet, 1992).

When other disciplines are involved in client care, it is imperative that all care provided is coordinated. Medical diagnoses are understood by all disciplines involved in client care; however, there also are problems of a nonmedical nature that are addressed by each discipline in a community setting. What nomenclature is used to communicate the nonmedical problems addressed? It is imperative that a common understanding of terminology used exists so that all disciplines can be working toward the same client goals.

In community health settings, many existing computer systems have emphasized the financial aspect of practice. The fact remains that there is a lack of systems that have done a good job of merging financial and clinical information. This problem has plagued information system users for a long time. In order to have meaningful reports for program planning, implementation, and evaluation, both financial and clinical data need to be addressed. Although many computer systems collect myriad statistical and financial data, most systems are difficult to use from a clinical standpoint. A system that emphasizes the financial and statistical components of a system may not be user-friendly for the practitioner and require that the practitioner document the same client data in several places within the software system. In summary, some computer software is not designed with nursing clinical practice in mind.

Other systems developed for community settings have emphasized the clinical aspects of care. In these systems, the practitioner has ease of entry with limited duplication. However, systems with this emphasis have typically had a more limited capability of producing management and financial reports that are useful to middle and senior managers. Systems that emphasize the clinical aspects of care permit the practitioner to enter client assessment data and outcomes easily, but these data are often not in a standardized format that permits the generation of reports that compile information about client progress or outcomes of groups of clients.

Newly developed information systems address the issue of incorporating both the financial and the clinical information in a single program. These systems enable the practitioner to enter client assessments and plans of care in a sequence that is logical to the practitioner. The results of care also are documented by a practitioner's single entry of data. Information is then moved to other forms and reports, eliminating multiple data entries on the part of the practitioner. From a management perspective, software that is capable of capturing and summarizing data in a useful format for management reports is a desired outcome of an information system.

Technology is now available that eliminates the need for a hard copy of the clinical record. Practitioners enter data regarding client assessment, care plans, and evaluation in hand-held computer terminals, which have the advantage of permitting data entry at the home or clinic site where nursing care is administered. Information from these hand-held computer terminals is then uploaded into a mainframe computer or file server via modem or docking port. This process makes client data immediately available to others who have use for the information. This technology has the potential to improve staff productivity and enhance communication among all users of client information, including care providers, office/billing staff, performance improvement/risk managers, and other managers.

In summary, information systems assist practitioners and managers to organize individual-level data from several sources and to facilitate communication among multiple users of the data. Data integration, practice guidance, and instant access to resource material are strengths of information systems for working with individual clients. Communication among multiple users of data, including nurse-to-nurse communication and interdisciplinary information exchange, are enhanced by information systems. Agency management also benefits from real-time information for both performance improvement activities and risk management. Problems encountered in the use of information systems for individual clients include lack of a common nomenclature for clear communication among nurses and members of other disciplines. In addition, problems arise in priorities between a clinical focus for information systems versus a financial focus.

MANAGING INFORMATION ABOUT POPULATION GROUPS

The second level of data systems describes population groups. Population groups consist of individuals who share issues or problems. For example, a population group may be as general as "newborn infants" or as specific as "newborn infants with a diagnosis of Down's syndrome." Information about client groups provides opportunities for comparison of data across practitioners, geographic locations, agencies, and communities.

As health care reform changes the health care delivery system, information about population groups is becoming more important. Payers are increasingly responsible for the entire continuum of care for a population group of "covered lives." As care delivery changes, information systems need to provide information that the new health care system demands. Information systems must capture data that will assess the effectiveness of care provided to groups of clients in a variety of community settings. These settings may be clients' residences, ambulatory care settings, schools, day care centers, or workplaces. Management needs information that tracks the outcomes of client care, processes used to achieve client outcomes, and the resources consumed in the process of obtaining the outcomes. Individual client information needs to be tracked across the continuum of care from wellness to death and across care settings as clients move from hospitals to home care to ambulatory settings and back again. Home and community health care that has traditionally generated income for an agency will move from a focus on income generation to being a cost center for large health care systems. In a capitated system where payers receive a flat monthly fee to care for a number of "covered lives," the impetus is for home care and community health services to be viewed as costs, because no additional revenue will be generated by providing these services. The ability to track costs and client outcomes and to use information to achieve efficiencies in care provision will be critical for, for example, contracting.

Comparison of statistical data among nurses is important. The types of data useful to share among nurses include information about client outcomes, processes used to achieve client outcomes, cost of care to achieve outcomes, and productivity. Description of the outcomes of client care in a community setting is imperative. As agencies compete for contracts in a managed care environment, the ability to demonstrate and document client outcomes is gaining increasing importance. Information systems can assist the agency in tracking and reporting outcomes. For example, one measure of client outcome is functional status. Staff at VNS rate a client's ability to perform Activities of Daily Living (ADL) and Instrumental Activities of Daily Living (IADL) on admission to service and upon discharge. If the client needed assistance with bathing on admission and was able to perform this function independently upon discharge, a positive outcome of care has been achieved. To view the agency's ability to achieve excellent client outcomes in client functional ability, it is necessary to group client outcome information. This information is useful for comparing internal agency outcomes over time as well as for comparing data among agencies. For example, suppose a fictitious agency identifies outcomes for clients who had a stroke and were dependent in bathing upon admission. In the first quarter of 1996, 25% of the agency's clients moved from being dependent in bathing upon admission to independent in bathing upon discharge, 26% in the second quarter, 28% in the third quarter, and 30% in the fourth quarter. There was a general upward trend in the ability of this agency to move clients toward independence in bathing after a stroke. Once such data are captured and organized, an agency can compare results over time and with other agencies. In the future, these kinds of reports will be important to agencies that wish to monitor progress toward obtaining excellent client outcomes.

The ability to compare statistical data among and between nurses is also important. If we follow the example of helping clients to become independent in bathing following a stroke, the next step is to determine what agency staff did to assist individual clients to achieve independence. Information systems must be able to help an agency determine not only what occurred in terms of client outcomes, but also the process used to achieve that outcome. Some examples follow:

- Which teaching materials were used by staff in working with the client?
- How was client education sequenced?
- What disciplines were involved in providing care to the client?
- Were physical and occupational therapy involved?
- Did the process used with clients who achieved independence differ from the process used with those who did not?

Properly designed information systems should be able to help an agency answer these questions about client outcomes.

A third aspect of data collection about groups of clients is the cost of achieving outcomes of care. Information systems should assist an agency in capturing data about the cost of providing care to clients. The number of home visits made to achieve client outcomes is a major component of the cost of care. The ability to achieve excellent client outcomes with a minimum number of visits is imperative. Alternative means of providing care also need to be considered in evaluating costs. It may be much less expensive for a client to come to the care provider for service, if the client is able, than to have a practitioner visit the home. If some or all of the care can be provided in an ambulatory, work, or school setting, costs can be decreased. Information systems provide management with the data needed to evaluate the effectiveness of various alternatives in care provision.

A fourth aspect of data collection includes information regarding agency resource allocation. Variation in cost may be due to the mixture and allocation of resources for clients. For example, one agency may use an LPN to perform less complex components of care such as frequent dressing changes; the registered nurse may assume responsibility for the more complex nursing functions, including periodic assessment and evaluation of the plan of care, case management, or care coordination functions. Differences in resource utilization may also be a factor in the mix of services provided to a client. For example, some agencies may use home care aides more intensively than others after a client is discharged from the hospital in the acute stages of illness. Once the client regains strength or some functional ability, the home care aide services are decreased. The hypothesis is that helping the client more intensively with personal care services during early convalescence conserves client strength so that teaching is more effective, thus enabling earlier discharge of the client from home care. Information systems that are designed to capture information about mix of services provided, process-related data, and allocation of agency resources provide valuable data for an agency. In a managed care environment, the success of home care will be not be measured by the number of visits made, but by how successful the agency is at moving the client toward independence, out of home care, into a less costly means of service delivery.

There are several challenges that are encountered in using information systems to capture data to demonstrate the effectiveness of care. These challenges occur within agencies as well as between agencies. One of the problems in comparing data among nurses, even in the same agency, is the lack of standardized classification schemes for client acuity. One nurse may be able to achieve an outcome such as the client's ability to perform a dressing change independently within five visits. Another nurse may achieve the same outcome as the first nurse but in eight visits. Does this mean that the second nurse is less skillful than the first nurse or does it mean that the there was a difference in client variables? The second nurse may have had a client with a more serious wound, or a client who had a functional limitation that made the dressing change more difficult. In fact, the nurse with the most visits may have been the most skilled, because he or she was able to teach a more complicated client in just eight visits. The lack of a standardized system for measuring acuity in community health has made this comparison more difficult.

As agencies attempt to measure the cost of achieving client outcomes, there are several problems that can occur. One of the problems with measurement is determining what indicator to use and being sure that the measurement has common meaning among practitioners and across agencies. For example, many agencies have a desire to compare staff productivity. As agencies become more concerned about the cost of providing care and achieving excellent client outcomes, productivity becomes increasingly important. High productivity translates into lower cost per visit. Because the home visit has become the accepted unit of service in home health care and community health, it is used for comparison between agencies. Productivity measures the number of home visits a nurse makes in a day. Even though the home visit has been the accepted unit of service for home care for a long period of time, there is no common formula for productivity computation, thus comparison across agencies becomes very difficult. For example, two agencies may have a common definition for a home visit, yet in computing staff productivity in number of home visits per day, each may use a different formula. One may count only visits that are billable to a funding source. Another may also count home visits that are made to evaluate a home care aide's plan of care but are not billable to a third-party source of funding. One agency may exclude hours that the nurse spends in agency meetings. Another may include those hours in the total time available for home visiting. One may include in-service meetings; another may exclude those hours. Thus, because there is not an accepted formula for computing home visits, comparison across agencies becomes very difficult.

In summary, information systems facilitate comparison of data within and between agencies. These comparisons assist an agency in determining effectiveness in achieving client outcomes, processes used to achieve excellent outcomes, cost of the outcomes obtained, and use of agency and community resources. Challenges encountered in comparison of data among agencies in a community setting include lack of a common method of identifying client acuity and lack of common definitions for accuracy in data comparisons.

DESCRIBING AND SHARING
COMMUNITY NEEDS AND SERVICES

At the community level, information systems are important in collecting, analyzing, and presenting health data regarding a community or communities. In a community setting, programs are developed to meet community needs, based upon a needs assessment. Community assessment data can be collected and organized in meaningful ways with the use of information systems. For example, demographic data, vital statistics information, and the results of surveys conducted at the community level may be available by census tract, zip code, city, or county. These data can be organized in an information system and presented with mapping software to give a comprehensive picture of the community's health status by census tract, zip code, city, or county. The ability to map data helps to pinpoint community problems such as census tracts with high numbers of low birth weight babies, tracts with large numbers of deaths due to cancer, or tracts with high numbers of teenage pregnancies.

Information about primary or secondary diagnoses for clients on an agency's caseload may also be organized by census tract or zip code. If vital statistic data can be overlaid for the same geographic areas, a picture emerges about the agency's current ability to meet community needs. For example, if the death rate from cancer is significantly higher in selected census tracts, the information system for an agency should be able to produce reports about the number of clients with a diagnosis of cancer who were served by the agency in those census tracts. If there are smaller-than-expected numbers of people with cancer diagnoses served by the agency in those census tracts, there are implications for program development or public relations.

A second use of information systems at the community level is in the area of program planning, implementation, and evaluation. For example, staff at VNS in Des Moines developed a teen pregnancy program in cooperation with the public school system. Community assessment data revealed that certain census tracts in the Des Moines area had higher-than-expected infant mortality rates. In those same census tracts there was a large number of teen births and low birth weight babies. Grant funding was sought on two fronts. One grant provided case management services in cooperation with public school nurses to clients who were in the school setting. A second grant provided case management services to teenagers who dropped out of the school system. Goals were set regarding teens' follow-through with prenatal care, persuading teens to quit smoking or quit using alcohol or drugs during pregnancy, follow-through with guidance and counseling provided by nurses, and securing appropriate nutrition. In addition, outcomes were tracked for teens. These outcomes included the trimester at which prenatal care began, number of low birth weight babies, and number of infant deaths. The information system captured data used to identify the processes used by staff in providing service (follow-through on teaching, referrals, nutrition counseling, prenatal appointments) and the outcomes of program implementation. The data were summarized on a quarterly basis and changes were made in the program based on the results of the data analysis.

Issues that arise for information system use and development at the community level include confidentiality of client information, lack of standardized language for describing services and outcomes, and collecting and analyzing data when several agencies are working together but have different software platforms. Assuring confidentiality of client information at the community level is important. In Des Moines, several agencies serve pregnant teens and provide a variety of services for this population. Agency staff identified that clients would benefit if there were information sharing among providers. Sharing of information provides an opportunity to ensure that the teens are getting the service each needs, to facilitate referrals among agencies, and to avoid duplication of services. Sharing of information would mean that teens would not need to repeat admission data for each agency to which they were referred for assistance. A coordinating committee with representatives from each agency met to determine the kinds of information it would be important to share. This group became known as Interchange. One of the major problems encountered by the group was how to maintain confidentiality of the information, yet have the information available when needed. Client permission for interagency sharing of data was obtained from each client upon admission to a participating agency. VNS became the repository of information for the coalition of agencies. An intake form was developed that included key demographic data and information about services each agency provides to the client, and problems the client had that could not be met by the admitting agency. Data are entered into the computer by VNS staff. Monthly and quarterly reports are generated for each participating Interchange agency. Reports include information about clients being served by each agency, the services being provided, and unmet needs. This has prevented duplication of effort as well as better coordination of services to clients.

The coordinating committee, known as the Interchange group, is now exploring the possibility of data entry and extraction by tying each agency into the VNS mainframe computer. The Management of Information System (MIS) staff at VNS can give different levels of security to users, depending on the level of access needed. For example, senior management has access to all levels within the computer, staff nurses have access to those files that pertain to client care, users within the Interchange group will have access to limited information and only for those client files served by the Interchange agencies. Interchange agencies will have access only to the individual client data essential for coordination of services.

A goal of Interchange is to have access to the information on-line as opposed to waiting for a computer report to be generated. A major hurdle to overcome to achieve this goal is that each agency has different software packages that are not compatible with each other. At this time, if an agency wants to go "live," on-line with the host computer, it must purchase the software—and in some cases hardware—that is compatible with the host computer. A computer platform that allows sharing of data among different computer software systems is desirable.

As agencies attempt to work together to assess community needs and solve community problems, the ability to have information systems that facilitate the sharing of information among agencies will become even more critical. As health care systems evolve that can provide a full continuum of client care from wellness programs to acute intensive care to home care and ambulatory care, the ability to track clients through the system will be imperative for providing good client care and ensuring excellent client outcomes to individual clients, to population groups, and to the community as a whole. The ability to collect and analyze data, ensure confidentiality of client information, determine the cost of achieving outcomes, and communicate that data to those who need it is essential.

CONCLUSIONS

Information systems have been used in community settings since the beginning of modern nursing. They have a tremendous capability of increasing an agency's effectiveness in providing service to individual clients, population groups, and communities. Information systems help agencies to organize data, evaluate the outcomes of services provided, compare and contrast the effectiveness of different approaches to service delivery, and standardize practice.

There are challenges to the use of data in information systems. These challenges include lack of a common nomenclature for staff in community settings to communicate clearly with each other. Lack of common definitions is a barrier to comparison of data among agencies. In addition, maintaining confidentiality of data becomes more of a challenge as information from a common database is shared among agencies. Finally, the variety of software platforms available to users today can present challenges in sharing common data files.

As changes in the health care system emerge, there are new opportunities and new challenges for providers. Information systems can assist organizations to collect, organize, and analyze data. The challenge will be to use that data effectively to provide excellent, cost-effective care to individuals, population groups, and communities.

REFERENCES

Martin, K. S., & Scheet, N. S. (1992). *The Omaha system: Applications for community health nursing.* Philadelphia: W. B. Saunders.

Stanhope, M., & Lancaster, J. (1992). *Community health nursing* (3rd ed.). St. Louis, MO: Mosby-Year Book.

SUPPORT BIBLIOGRAPHY

I. OVERVIEW OF NURSING INFORMATICS

Adaskin, E. J., Hughes, L., McMullan, P., McLean, M., & McMorris, D. (1994). The impact of computerization on nursing: An interview study of users and facilitators. *Computers in Nursing, 12*(3), 141-148.

American Nurses Association. (1994). *The scope of practice for nursing informatics.* Washington, DC: Author.

American Nurses Association. (1995). *Standards of practice for nursing informatics.* Washington, DC: Author.

American Nurses Association. (1997). *Nursing Information and Data Set Evaluation Center (NID-SEC): Standards and scoring guidelines.* Washington, DC: Author.

American Organization of Nurse Executives. (1994). Influencing healthcare informatics. *Nursing Management, 25*(7), 31.

Anderson, B. (1992). Nursing informatics: Career opportunities inside and out. *Computers in Nursing, 10*(4), 165-170.

Blois, M. (1987). What is it that computers compute? *Clinical Computing, 4*(3), 31-33, 56.

Brunner, B. K. (1993). Health care-oriented telecommunications: The wave of the future. *Topics in Health Information Management, 14*(1), 54-61.

Cassey, M. Z., Kane, W. P., & Sutton, L. S. (1993). On-line access to nursing literature. *Computers in Nursing, 11*(5), 230-235.

Graves, J., & Corcoran, S. (1989). The study of nursing informatics. *Image: Journal of Nursing Scholarship, 21*(4), 227-231.

Hays, B. J., Norris, J., Martin, K. S., & Androwich, I. (1994). Informatics issues for nursing's future. *Advances in Nursing Science, 16*(4), 71-81.

Heller, B., Damrosch, S., Romano, C., & McCarthy, M. (1989). Graduate specialization in nursing informatics. *Computers in Nursing, 7*(2), 68-76.

Kuhn, T. (1970). *The structure of scientific revolutions.* Chicago: University of Chicago Press.

Maher, M. P. (1994). The CNS and nursing informatics. *Clinical Nurse Specialist, 8*(2), 103-108.

Meyrowitz, J. (1995). *No sense of place: The impact of electronic media on social behavior.* New York: Oxford University Press.

Stone, A. (1995). *The war of desire and technology at the close of the mechanical age.* Cambridge, MA: MIT Press.

Werley, H., & Lang, N. (Eds.). (1988). *Identification of the Nursing Minimum Data Set.* New York: Springer.

II. HEALTH INFORMATION SYSTEMS

Andrew, W. F. (1994). New technologies mean a cable-free future for point-of-care. *HealthCare Informatics*, *11*(5), 33-34, 36-44.

Andrew, W. F. (1994). Point-of-care technology: The window into the integrated clinical database, part 9. *Computers in Nursing*, *12*(3), 171-173.

Andrew, W. F. (1994). Point-of-care technology: The window into the integrated clinical database, part 10. *Computers in Nursing*, *12*(4), 210-212.

Aydin, C. E. (1994). Professional agendas and computer-based patient records: Negotiating for control. *Topics in Health Information Management*, *15*(1), 41-51.

Bauer, A. (1992). AHA study defines bedside terminal issues. *Healthcare Informatics*, *5*, 74-79.

Cella, D. F., & Lloyd, S. R. (1994). Data collection for patient-reported information. *Quality Management in Health Care*, *2*(4), 28-35.

Dassenko, D. (1993, August). Vendor partnering yields progress toward the computerized patient record. *Healthcare Informatics*, pp. 30, 32.

Dawe, U., Warnock-Matherton, A., & Ross, S. (1993). Mapping the future of hospital information systems: Priorities for nursing applications. *Computers in Nursing*, *11*(2), 61-66.

Gittleman, M. (1992, November). Paperless by 2000: Implementing EDI for healthcare claims processing. *Healthcare Informatics*, pp. 86-87.

Gleason, B. (1993). Rural hospitals set the pace for computerized documentation. *Nursing Management*, *24*(7), 49-50.

Gobis, L. J. (1994). Computerized patient records: Start preparing now. *Journal of Nursing Administration*, *24*(9), 15-16, 60.

Golob, R. (1994). Securing a bridge to the CPR: Clinical data repositories. *Healthcare Informatics*, *11*(2), 50-58.

Herrick, K. M., & McCullough, S. (1989). Introducing nurses to computers in a multi-hospital environment. *Nursing Management*, *20*(7), 31-34.

Laureto-Ward, R., & Cooper Weidner, C. (1993). Poised for change: Installing an enterprise-wide MIS. *Healthcare Informatics*, *10*(9), 24-26.

Martin, G., & Baker, G. (1993, May). Measuring the benefits of bedside systems. *Healthcare Informatics*, pp. 26-30.

Morrissey, J. (1994, October 10). Workstations that work. *Modern Healthcare*, pp. 40-44.

Nauright, L. P., & Simpson, R. L. (1994). Benefits of hospital information systems as seen by front-line nurses and general hospital staff. *Journal of Nursing Administration*, *24*(Suppl. 4), 26-32.

Pulliam, L., Valentine, J., Raymond, J., & Racine, D. (1992). Implementation of a computerized information system in a long-term care facility. *Computers in Nursing*, *10*(5), 201-207.

Rheinecker, P. (1993). Strategies for successful information system development. *Health Progress*, *74*(6), 18-21, 26.

Rollins, S. (1994, May). Technology on the move: Eliminating paper at the point of care. *Healthcare Informatics*, pp. 58-62.

Seufert, J. (1993). A vision of clinical informatics. *The Journal of the Healthcare Information and Management Systems Society*, *7*(4), 5-10.

Simpson, R. (1991). Electronic patient charts: Beware the hype. *Nursing Management*, *22*(4), 13-14.

Simpson, R. L. (1994). How technology can encourage collaborative practice. *Nursing Administration Quarterly*, *18*(4), 79-83.

Slivka, S. K., Roberts, D. L., & Pryor, T. A. (1993). Information systems: A technology to implement process redesign. *Journal of the Society for Health Systems*, *4*(1), 55-64.

Staggers, N., & Mills, M. E. (1994). Nurse-computer interaction: Staff performance outcomes. *Nursing Research*, *43*(3), 144-150.

Steiniger, V. (1994, October). Checklist helps C-R-E-A-T-E a successful CPR. *Health Management Technology*, pp. 37-42.

Tan, J. K. H., & Hanna, J. (1994). Integrating health care with information technology: Knitting patient information through networking. *Health Care Management Review, 19*(2), 72-80.

Tarte, J. P., & Bogiages, C. C. (1992, February). Patient-centered care delivery and the role of information systems. *Computers in Healthcare*, pp. 44-46.

Wilson, D., Nelson, N. C., Rosebrock, B. J., Hujcs, M. T., Wilner, D. G., & Buxton, R. B. (1994). Using an integrated point of care system: A nursing perspective. *Topics in Health Information Management, 14*(4), 24-29.

III. CLINICAL NURSING INFORMATION SYSTEMS

Amann, M. C. (1994). Informatics: The application to occupational health nursing. *American Association of Occupational Health Nurses' Journal, 42*(8), 391-396.

Baldwin, L., & McGinnis, C. (1994). A computer-generated shift report. *Nursing Management, 25*(9), 61-64.

Berg, C. M., & Gould, W. (1991). Patient care systems: Do they meet the needs of nursing? *Computers in Healthcare, 12*(4), 26, 30, 32.

Bradley, V. (1994). Innovative informatics: Our computerized patient-tracking system. *Journal of Emergency Nursing, 20*(4), 320-323.

Braunstein, M. L. (1994). Electronic patient records for homecare nursing. *Computers in Nursing, 12*(5), 232-238.

Bursley, H., Tikkamen, P., Feistrizer, N., Zweber, M., & Murdock, D. (1985). Hospital information systems: The relationship between nurse involvement in selection and nurse utilization. *Journal of Medical Systems, 9*(1/2), 19-27.

Chu, S. (1993). Clinical information systems: A fourth generation. Part I. *Nursing Management, 24*(10), 59-60.

Chu, S. (1993). Clinical information systems: The nursing interface. Part II. *Nursing Management, 24*(11), 58-60.

Cooper, M. C. (1993). The intersection of technology and care in the ICU. *Advances in Nursing Science, 15*(3), 23-32.

Cooper, M. C. (1994). Care: Antidote for nurses' love-hate relationship with technology. *American Journal of Critical Care, 3*(5), 402-403.

Couillard-Getreuer, D. (1993). Informatics and information in nursing. *Current Issues in Cancer Nursing Practice, 2*(1), 1-11.

Frick, T., Rein, A., & Parks, V. (1993). Benefits of an automated narcotic retrieval system. *Nursing Management, 24*(7), 57-59.

Girgenti, J. R., & Mathis, A. C. (1994). Putting psychiatric nursing standards into clinical practice. *Journal of Psychosocial Nursing, 32*(6), 39-42.

Graves, J., & Corcoran, S. (1988). Design of nursing information systems. Conceptual and practice elements. *Journal of Professional Nursing, 4*(3), 168-177.

Haberman, M. L., & Swenson, G. N. (1993). Enhancing professional communication: A formal computerized nurse-to-nurse consultation system. *Nursing Administration Quarterly, 18*(1), 66-79.

Harnisch, P., Honan, S., & Torkelson, R. (1993). Quality improvement approach to nursing care planning: Implementing practical computerized standards. *Journal for Healthcare Quality, 15*(5), 6-13.

Hettinger, B., & Brazile, R. (1992). A database design for community health data. *Computers in Nursing, 10*(3), 109-115.

Katz, J., & Schroeder, P. (1994). Linking key functions and important aspects of care: Perspectives on preoperative, medical-surgical, and prenatal nursing. *Journal of Nursing Care Quality, 9*(1), 66-77.

Lancaster, L. (1993). Nursing information systems in the year 2000: Another perspective. *Computers in Nursing, 11*(1), 3-5.

Matteson, P. S., & Hawkins, J. W. (1993). Facilitating the nurse practitioner's research role: Using a microcomputer for data entry in clinical settings. *Journal of the American Academy of Nurse Practitioners, 5*(3), 125-129.

Meikle, S. M. (1994, January-February). The computer-oriented paperless operating room. *Today's O.R. Nurse.*

Nicol, S. T., & Dyle, J. A. (1993). Innovations in anesthesia pre-screening through data systems and telecommunications. *The Journal of the Healthcare Information and Management Systems Society, 7*(4), 33-38.

Ozbolt, J., & Grave, J. R. (1993). Clinical nursing informatics: Developing tools for knowledge workers. *Advances in Clinical Nursing Research,* 409-429.

Paganelli, B. (1989). Criteria for the selection of a bedside information system for acute care units. *Computers in Nursing, 7*(5), 214-221.

Patterson, C. (1991). New Joint Commission standards for 1991 require RN decision making. *Nursing Administration Quarterly, 15*(4), 65-68.

Potthoff, S. J., Kane, R. L., Bartlett, J., & McKee, A. S. (1994). Developing a managed care clinical information system to assess outcomes of substance abuse treatment. *Clinical Performance and Quality Healthcare, 2*(3), 148-153.

Ripich, S., Morre, S., & Breuman, P. (1992). A new nursing median: Computer networks for group intervention. *Journal of Psychosocial Nursing Mental Health Service, 30*(7), 15-20.

Schroder, M. (1987). Computers in nursing: Applications in ambulatory care. *Nursing Economics, 5*(1), 27-31.

Schroeder, M. A., & Carter, J. (1989). Development of a database management system for an obstetrics unit. *Computers in Nursing, 7*(3), 112-118.

Simpson, R. L. (1994). The computer-based patient record and how it will affect the nurse's practice. In J. McCloskey & H. Grace (Eds.), *Current issues in nursing* (4th ed., pp. 270-275). St. Louis, MO: C. V. Mosby.

Simpson, R. L. (1994). Computer networks show great promise in supporting AIDS patients. *Nursing Administration Quarterly, 18*(2), 92-95.

Trofino, J. (1993). Voice-activated nursing documentation: On the cutting edge. *Nursing Management, 24*(7), 28-33.

Turley, J. (1992). A framework for the transition from nursing record to a nursing information system. *Nursing Outlook, 40*(4), 177-181.

Zielstorff, R., Jette, A., & Barnett, G. (1990). Issues in designing an automated record system for clinical care and research. *Advanced in Nursing Science, 13*(2), 75-88.

IV. NURSING ADMINISTRATION
AND MANAGEMENT INFORMATION SYSTEMS

Barry, T. L. (1994). Computer support for continuous quality improvement. *Journal for Healthcare Quality, 16*(2), 16-17, 40.

Cassidy, B., Dowell, S., & Bloomrosen, M. (1992, April). Health information management: Better care through quality data. *Computers in Healthcare,* pp. 37-42.

Chen, J., & Yeung, T. W. (1993). Hybrid expert-system approach to nurse scheduling. *Computers in Nursing, 11*(4), 183-190.

Custer, M. L. (1993). Enhancing case management through computerized patient files. *Clinical Nurse Specialist, 7,* 141-147.

Delaney, C., & Huber, D. (1996). *A Nursing Management Minimum Data Set (NMMDS): A report of an invitational conference.* Chicago: American Organization of Nurse Executives.

Edwardson, S., & Grovannetti, P. (1987). A review of cost-accounting methods for nursing services. *Nursing Economics, 5,* 107-117.

Finnegan, S. A., Abel, M., Dobler, T., Hudon, L., & Terry, B. (1993). Automated patient acuity: Linking nursing systems and quality measurement with patient outcomes. *Journal of Nursing Administration, 23*(5), 62-71.

Fralic, M. (1984, December). Using a PERT planning network to manage a nursing service computer system installation. *Journal of Nursing Administration,* pp. 29-31.

Fralic, M. F. (1989). Decision support systems: Essential for quality administrative decisions. *Nursing Administration Quarterly, 14*(1), 1-8.

Grinde, T. (1994). Implementing a nursing administration local area network. *Nursing Management, 25*(7), 36-37.

Hendrickson, G., & Kovner, C. T. (1990). Effects of computers on nursing resource use. *Computers in Nursing, 8*(1), 16-22.

Hlusko, D. L., Weatherly, K. S., Franklin, K. G., Wallace, S., & Williamson, S. (1994). Computerization of a nursing financial management system using continuous quality improvement as a framework. *Computers in Nursing, 12*(4), 193-200.

Huber, D. G., Delaney, C., Crossley, J., Mehmert, M., & Ellerbe, S. (1992). A Nursing Management Minimum Data Set. *Journal of Nursing Administration, 22*(7/8), 35-39.

Pulliam, L., & McNulty, S. L. (1992). Computerized quality assurance monitoring: A collaborative project. *Journal of Nursing Care Quality, 7*(1), 44-52.

Schwanitz, L. (1993). Automation controls inventory, cuts costs. *OR Manager, 9*(7), 16-17.

Schyve, P. M., & Kamowski, D. B. (1994). Information management and quality improvement: The Joint Commission's perspective. *Quality Management in Health Care, 2*(4), 54-62.

Seiter, T. J., & Pagnotta, R. R. (1994, June). It's a jungle out there: Strategies for controlling information systems costs. *Healthcare Financial Management,* pp. 41-46.

Siroky, K. A., & Fields, W. L. (1992). Automated data entry and analysis for unit-based quality assurance programs. *Journal of Nursing Quality Care, 7*(1), 35-43.

V. STANDARDIZED DATABASES

Agency for Health Care Policy and Research. (1991). *Report to Congress: The feasibility of linking research-related data bases to federal medical administrative data bases* (AHCPR Pub. No. 91-0003). Washington, DC: Government Printing Office.

Burns, C. (1993). Using a comprehensive taxonomy of diagnoses to describe the practice of pediatric nurse practitioners: Findings of a field study. *Journal of Pediatric Health Care, 7*(3), 115-121.

Carter, J. H., Moorhead, S. A., McCloskey, J. C., & Bulechek, G. M. (1995). Using the nursing interventions classification to implement Agency for Health Care Policy and Research guidelines. *Journal of Nursing Care Quality, 9*(2), 76-86.

Daly, J. M., McCloskey, J. C., & Bulechek, G. M. (1994). Nursing interventions classification use in longterm care. *Geriatric Nursing, 15*(1), 41-46.

Delaney, C., & Huber, D. (1996). *A Nursing Management Minimum Data Set (NMMDS): A report of an invitational conference.* Chicago: American Organization of Nurse Executives.

Delaney, C., & Mehmert, P. (1990). Electronic transfer of clinical NMDS facilitates nursing diagnoses validation. In *Proceedings of the Fourteenth Annual Symposium on Computer Applications in Medical Care (SCAMC).* Washington, DC: IEEE Computer Society Press.

Delaney, C., & Mehmert, P. (1991). Utility of NMDS is validation of computerized nursing diagnoses. In R. Carroll-Johnson (Ed.), *Classification of nursing diagnoses: Proceedings of the Ninth Annual North American Nursing Diagnosis Association.* Philadelphia: J. B. Lippincott.

Delaney, C., Mehmert, P., Prophet, C., Bellinger, S. R., Huber, D. G., & Ellerbe, S. (1992). Standardized nursing language for healthcare information systems. *Journal of Medical Systems, 16*(4), 145-159.

Giovannetti, P. (1987). Implications of the Nursing Minimum Data Set. In K. Hannak, M. Reimer, W. C. Mills, & S. Letourneau (Eds.), *Clinical judgement and decision making: The future with nursing diagnosis* (pp. 552-555). New York: John Wiley.

Grobe, S. J. (1990). Nursing intervention lexicon and taxonomy study: Language and classification methods. *Advances in Nursing Science, 13,* 22-33.

Halloran, E. J. (1988). Conceptual consideration, decision criteria and guidelines for the Nursing Minimum Data Set from an administrative perspective. In H. H. Werley & N. M. Lang (Eds.), *Identification of the Nursing Minimum Data Set* (pp. 48-66). New York: Springer.

Henry, S. B, Holzemer, W. L., Reilly, C. A., & Campbell, K. E. (1994). Terms used by nurses to describe patient problems: Can SNOMED III represent nursing concepts in the patient record. *Journal of the American Medical Informatics Association, 1*(1), 61-74.

Hettinger, B. J., & Brazile, R. P. (1994). Health level seven (HL7): Standard for healthcare electronic data transmissions. *Computers in Nursing, 12*(1), 13-16.

Iowa Outcomes Project. (1997). *Nursing outcomes classification* (NOC) (M. Johnson & M. Maas, Eds.). St. Louis, MO: C. V. Mosby.

Lee, F. W. (1992). Using database software for quantitative review and active caseload lists in a community health setting. *Topics in Health Information Management, 13*(1), 35-44.

Leske, J. S., & Werley, H. H. (1992). Use of the Nursing Minimum Data Set. *Computers in Nursing, 10*(6), 259-263.

Martin, K. S., & Scheet, N. J. (1992). *The Omaha system: Applications for community health nursing.* Philadelphia: W. B. Saunders.

McCloskey, J. C., & Bulechek, G. M. (1995). *Nursing interventions classification* (2nd ed.). St. Louis, MO: Mosby-Year Book.

McCormick, K. A. (1988). A unified nursing language system. In M. J. Ball, K. J. Hannah, U. Gerdin Helger, & H. Peterson (Eds.), *Nursing informatics: Where caring and technology meet* (pp. 168-178). New York: Springer.

McLane, A. M. (1987). Measurement and validation of diagnostic concepts: A decade of progress. *Heart & Lung, 16*(pt. 1), 616-624.

McPhillips, R. (1988). Essential elements for the Nursing Minimum Data Set as seen by federal officials. In H. H. Werley & N. M. Lang (Eds.), *Identification of the Nursing Minimum Data Set* (pp. 325-333). New York: Springer.

Mehmert, P., & Delaney, C. (1991). Validation of defining characteristics of immobility using the computerized NMDS. *Nursing Diagnosis, 2*(4), 143-154.

Mehmert, P. A., Delaney, C., Crossley, J., & Prophet, C. (1992). Validation of nursing diagnosis: Clinical and management applications. *Nursing Management, 20*(7), 24-26, 28, 30.

North American Nursing Diagnosis Association. (1996). *North American Nursing Diagnosis Association: Taxonomy I: 1996-97.* St. Louis, MO: Author.

Ozbolt, J. G., Fruchtnicht, J. N., & Hayden, J. R. (1994). Toward data standards for clinical nursing information. *Journal of the American Medical Informatics Association, 1*(2), 175-185.

Rios, H., Delaney, C., Kruckeberg, T., Chung, Y., & Mehmert, P. A. (1991). Validation of defining characteristics of four nursing diagnoses using a computerized data base. *Journal of Professional Nursing, 7,* 293-299.

Rittman, M. R., & Gorman, R. H. (1992). Computerized databases: Privacy issues in the development of the Nursing Minimum Data Set. *Computers in Nursing, 10*(1), 14-18.

Ryan, P., & Delaney, C. (1995). Nursing Minimum Data Set. In J. J. Fitzpatrick & J. S. Stevenson (Eds.), *Annual review of nursing research* (pp. 169-194). New York: Springer.

Werley, H. H., & Lang, N. M. (1988). *Identification of the Nursing Minimum Data Set.* New York: Springer.

Williams, C. (1991). The Nursing Minimum Data Set: A major priority for public health nursing but not a panacea. *American Journal of Public Health, 81*(4), 413-414.

VI. COMPUTER ASSISTED DECISION MAKING

Artificial Intelligence: Expert Systems

Bobis, K., & Bachand, P. (1993). Expert systems: The nurses' toolbox. *Nursing Management, 24*(7), 103-104.

Franco, A., Farr, F. L., King, J. D., Clark, J. S., & Haug, P. J. (1990). "NEONATE": An expert application for the "HELP" system: Comparison of the computer's and the physician's problem list. *Journal of Medical Systems, 14*(5), 297-306.

Harding, W. T., Redmond, R. T., & Corley, M. C. (1993). Loading a nursing expert system from text: A case study. *Computers in Nursing, 11*(6), 277-281.

Hoesing, H., Cuddigan, J., & Logan, S. (1990). COMMES. Using a computerized consultant in professional practice. In G. G. Mayer et al. (Eds.), *Patient care delivery models.* Rockville, MD: Aspen.

Lauri, S. (1992). Using a computer simulation program to assess the decision-making process in child health care. *Computers in Nursing, 10*(4), 171-177.

Schank, M. (1988). The potential of expert systems in nursing. *Journal of Nursing Administration, 18*(6), 26-32, 237, 1297-1298.

Taylor, T. R. (1990). The computer and clinical decision-support systems in primary care. *The Journal of Family Practice, 30*(2), 137-149.

Thompson, C. B., Ryan, S. A., & Kitzman, H. (1990). Expertise: The basis for expert system development. *Advances in Nursing Science, 13*(2), 1-10.

Woolery, L. (1990). Expert nurses and expert systems. *Computers in Nursing, 8*(1), 23-28.

VII. COMPUTERS AND RESEARCH

Barnsteiner, J. H. (1993, Spring). The online journal of knowledge synthesis for nursing. *Reflections,* p. 8.

Bear, G. C., Richards, H. C., & Lancaster, P. (1987). Attitudes toward computers: Validation of a computer attitudes scale. *Journal of Educational Computing Research, 3*(2), 207-218.

Lange, L. L., & Jacox, A. (1993). Using large data bases in nursing and health policy research. *Journal of Professional Nursing, 9*(4), 204-211.

Moritz, P. (1990). Information technology: A priority for nursing research. *Computers in Nursing, 8*(3), 111-115.

Murphy, C. A., Maynard, M., & Morgan, G. (1994). Pretest and post-test attitudes of nursing personnel toward a patient care information system. *Computers in Nursing, 12*(5), 239-244.

Stonge, J., & Brodt, A. (1985). Assessment of nurses' attitudes toward computerization. *Computers in Nursing, 3*(4), 154-158.

Zielstorff, R., Abrahamo, I., Werley, H., Saba, V., & Schwirian, P. (1989). Guidelines for reporting innovations in computer based information systems for nursing. *Computers in Nursing, 7*(5), 203-208.

VIII. LEGALITIES, ETHICS, AND POLICY

Agich, G. J. (1994). Privacy and medical record information. *Journal of the American Medical Informatics Association, 1*(4), 323-324.

Baumgart, A. J. (1993). Quality through health policy: The Canadian example. *International Nursing Review, 40*(6), 167-170.

Bialorucki, T., & Blaine, M. J. (1992). Protecting patient confidentiality in the pursuit of the ultimate computerized information system. *Journal of Nursing Care Quality, 7*(1), 53-56.

Brennan, P. F. (1987). Smart cards & networks: Promote access to information. *Today's OR Nurse, 9*(7), 23-27.

Butzen, F., & Furler, F. (1986). Computer security: A necessary element of integrated information systems. *Bulletin of the Medical Library Association, 74*(3), 210-216.

Cavazos, E., & Morin, G. (1995). *Cyber space and the law.* Cambridge, MA: MIT Press.

Congressional Office of Technology Assessment. (1994). Emerging threats to privacy: Computers and your health care records. *Consumer Research Magazine, 77,* 33-36.

Cross, M. (1995, October). Keeping records private: Encryption offers the best hope for maintaining the privacy of clinical information transmitted on the Internet. *Health Data Management,* pp. 18-20.

Curran, M., & Curran, K. (1991). The ethics of information. *Journal of Nursing Administration, 21*(1), 47-49.

Faaoso, N. (1992). Automated patient care systems: The ethical impact. *Nursing Management, 23*(7), 46-48.

Gardner, R. M. (1994). Integrated computerized records provide improved quality of care with little loss of privacy. *Journal of the American Medical Informatics Association, 1*(4), 320-322.

Gellman, R. (1995, January-February). Fair health information practices. *Behavioral Healthcare Tomorrow,* pp. 65-68.

Fishman, D. (1994). Confidentiality. *Computers in Nursing, 12*(2), 73-77.

Lindell, A. R. (1987, March-April). Piracy: Pirate or privateer. *Journal of Professional Nursing,* pp. 78, 124.

Millholland, D. K. (1994). Privacy and confidentiality of patient information. *Journal of Nursing Administration, 24*(2), 19-24.

Nicoll, L. H. (1994). Modern day pirates: Software users and abusers. *Journal of Nursing Administration, 24*(1), 18-20.

Patrikas, E. O. (1993). Electronic databases and privacy protection: Issues for a free society. *Topics in Health Information Management, 14*(1), 62-68.

Petrucci, K. E., & Petrucci, P. A. (1991). Nursing technology. *Nursing Economics, 9*(3), 188-190.

Sieracki, C. A. (1993). Organizational liability prevention: Automated profiles. *Nursing Management, 24*(7), 60-64.

Simpson, R. L. (1994). Ensuring patient data privacy, confidentiality and security. *Nursing Management, 25*(7), 18-20.

Simpson, R. L. (1995). Ethics in the information age. *Nursing Management, 26*(11), 20-21.

Simpson, R. L. (1995). How will state-level reforms affect your information systems? *Nursing Management, 26*(5), 20-21.

Talob, R. (1994). Copyright, legal, and ethical issues in the Internet environment. *Tech Trends, 39*(2), 11-14.

Thuraisingham, B. (1991, Winter). The inference problem in database security. *Cipher,* pp. 51-60.

Tufle, E. (1974). *Data analysis for politic and policy.* Englewood Cliffs, NJ: Prentice Hall.

Waller, A. A., & Fulton, D. K. (1993). The electronic chart: Keeping it confidential and secure. *Journal of Health and Hospital Law, 26*(4), 104-109.

White, N. (1992). Working with display screen equipment. *Occupational Health, 44*(4), 111-113.

Woolery, L. K. (1990). Professional standards and ethical dilemmas in nursing information systems. *Journal of Nursing Administration, 20*(10), 50-53.

IX. GLOBAL RESOURCES/INTERNET/VIRTUAL NURSING

Alva, D. (1994, July). WANs all over this LAN. *Healthcare Informatics,* pp. 38-42.

Ayre, R. (1994, October 11). Making the Internet connection. *PC Magazine,* pp. 118-184.

Bank, D. (1994, September 11). IBM, Home Shopping Network boost their Internet ties. *Waterloo Courier*, pp. B1-B2.

Bennett, V. M. (1994). Electronic document delivery using the Internet. *Bulletin of the Medical Library Association*, *82*(2), 163-167.

Benson, J. (1994, August). Searching for stock photos on-line. *Macworld*, pp. 124-127.

Bott, E., & Lipkis, T. (1994, September). The net result. *PC Computing*, pp. 122-169.

Brandt, R., & Cortese, A. (1994, June 27). Bill Gates' vision. *Business Week*, pp. 56-60.

Brauman, J. I., Voss, D. F., & Appenzeller. (1994). Computing: Networks and modeling [Editorial]. *Science*, *265*, 851.

Bruckman, A., Dertouzos, M., Domnitz, R., Felde, N., Kapor, M., Roetter, M., & Schrage, M. (1994, August/September). Seven thinkers in search of an information highway. *Technology Review*, pp. 42-52.

Cefola, R. N. (1994). The Internet. *Hospital Pharmacy*, *29*, 727-728.

Chapman, R. H., Reiley, P., McKinney, J., Welch, K., Toomey, B., & McCausland, M. (1994). Implementing a local area network for nursing in a large teaching hospital. *Computers in Nursing*, *12*(2), 82-88.

Churbuck, D. C. (1993, November 22). On the electronic frontier. *Forbes*, pp. 170-171.

Clark, D. (1994, September 19). Group of companies, agencies to test rapid transmission of medical images. *Wall Street Journal*.

Clement, G. P. (1994, September). Library without walls. *Internet World*, pp. 60-64.

Dykeman, J. (1994). Global technology: Small world, big job. *Beyond Computing*, *3*(5), 35-38.

Glowniak, J. V., & Bushway, M. K. (1994). Computer networks as a medical resource: Accessing and using the Internet. *Journal of the American Medical Association*, *271*(24), 1934-1939.

Graves, J. R. (1994, Fall). Library updates. *Reflections*, p. 39.

Hauptman, R., & Motin, S. (1994). The Internet, cyberethics, and virtual morality. *Online*, *18*(2), 8-9.

Kalin, S. W., & Tennant, R. (1991). Beyond OPACS . . . The wealth of information resources on the Internet. *Database*, *14*(4), 28-33.

Miller, M. J. (1994, October 11). Bill Gates ponders the Internet. *PC Magazine*, p. 79.

Morrison, D. (1994). Users declare a truce in the operating systems war. *Beyond Computing*, *3*(5), 27-28, 33.

Nicastro, L. (1993, August). The Internet goes to the head of the class. *Network Computing*, pp. 28-29.

Nicoll, L. H. (1993). Accessing literature. *Journal of Nursing Administration*, *23*(6), 7-8, 15.

Nicoll, L. H. (1994). An introduction to the Internet Part I: History, structure, and access. *Journal of Nursing Administration*, *24*(3), 9-11.

Nicoll, L. H. (1994). An intro to the Internet Part II: Addresses and resources. *Journal of Nursing Administration*, *24*(5), 11-13, 59.

Nicoll, L. H. (1994). An intro to the Internet Part III: The Internet and other online services. *Journal of Nursing Administration*, *24*(7/8), 15-17.

Nicoll, L. H. (1994). Modern day pirates: Software users and abusers. *Journal of Nursing Management*, *24*(1), 18-20.

Schneider, D. (1993, Spring). Internet: Linking nurses, scholars, libraries. *Reflections*, p. 9.

Sparks, S. (1993). Electronic networking for nurses. *Image: Journal of Nursing Scholarship*, *25*(3), 245-248.

Taira, F. (1993). Driving down the electronic highway. *Computers in Nursing*, *11*(5), 219-221.

Valiant, S., & Rosenberg, R. (1993). Evolving private networks in Europe. *Telecommunications*, *27*(2), 28-33.

Waldrop, M. M. (1994). Software agents prepare to sift the riches of cyberspace. *Science*, *265*, 882-883.

Author Index

Subject Index

About the Chairperson
and Editors

Diane Huber, PhD, RN, FAAN, is an Associate Professor, College of Nursing, University of Iowa, where she is one of the core faculty in Nursing Service Administration teaching both graduate and undergraduate students. She specializes in leadership and nursing care management. She also is the Adjunct Director of Nursing at Mercy Hospital, Iowa City, Iowa. This adjunct position is a service-education collaborative position. She is active in a variety of professional nursing organizations, especially the American Organization of Nurse Executives and the American Nurses Association. Huber has held nursing positions in ambulatory care and acute care. She has been a staff nurse, nurse supervisor, and division director. Her clinical specialty is maternal-child nursing with an emphasis on pediatrics and intensive care nursing. Her research areas are: human resources management, nursing administration, and informatics applications, especially a Nursing Management Minimum Data Set and a Management Innovations Evaluation portfolio; and second: maternal-child nursing, especially fatigue in postpartum women. Her most recent research projects are related to the use of nurse extenders, the development and testing of a nursing management minimum data set, a survey of nursing centers, and post-operative vital signs monitoring. She has received the American Nurses' Foundation/American Organization of Nurse Executives' Scholar award (1991), and the 1994 American Organization of Nurse Executives' Research Scholar Award. She has been involved with 15 funded projects, has authored one book, has over 30 publications, and has done numerous international, national, and local presentations of her work.

Sue Moorhead, PhD, RN, is an Assistant Professor at the University of Iowa College of Nursing. She teaches an overview of nursing course for beginning nursing students. She also supervises senior students in internship experiences during the final clinical course. In addition, she is a Colonel in the U.S. Army Reserve, with both active duty and reserve experience. Most recently, she completed assignments as chief nurse in the two U.S. Army reserve hospitals in Iowa. Her research interests focus on the development and implementation of standardized nursing language. She is an investigator on the Nursing Interventions Classification (NIC) team and has developed nursing interventions in the classification. She presently serves as the facilitator for the testing of this classification at Genesis Medical Center in Davenport, Iowa as part of the current grant. In addition, Moorhead is an investigator on the Nursing Outcomes Classification (NOC) and chairs the group developing outcomes in the psychological/cognitive area. Her current research focuses on mapping non-standardized nursing data into standardized language using these classifications. In addition, she works with nurses attempting to add standardized languages in both practice and educational settings. She has been a board member for several years; this is the second volume she has edited.

Connie Delaney, PhD, RN, is an Associate Professor in the College of Nursing, University of Iowa, where she teaches nursing informatics at the master's and doctoral levels. She is an adjunct Associate Professor in the School of Library and Information Science and has an adjunct staff position in nursing informatics at the University of Iowa Hospital. She is PI or Co-PI of three research teams that focus on standardized language development and large database research: the Nursing Diagnosis Extension & Classification Research Team (NDEC), representing a collaborative effort with the North American Nursing Diagnosis Association (NANDA); the Nursing Management Minimum Data Set (NMMDS) Research Team, a collaborative effort with the American Organization of Nurse Executives; and the Nursing Minimum Data Set (NMDS) research team, representing a collaborative effort among more than 10 national sites to advance development of methodologies and use of the NMDS. She is a member of multiple professional associations related to nursing, informatics, and administration. Most recently she served at the American Nurses Association to establish the National Information & Data Set Evaluation Center (NIDSEC). Delaney is active in statewide health care reform and development of statewide information systems and in numerous national information system initiations. She serves on the Steering Committee for the National Library of Medicine-funded initiative at the University of Iowa, Integrated Advanced Information Management System (IAIMS).

About the Contributors

Charlene Allred, PhD, RN, is Program Director for Nursing Systems Administration, School of Nursing, Duke University.

Gary Bargstadt, MBA, MS, RN, is President, Visiting Nurse Services, Des Moines, Iowa.

Julia G. Behrenbeck, MS, MPH, RN, is with Information Services, Mayo Medical Center.

Susan A. Briske, BS, RN, is with the Department of Nursing, Mayo Medical Center.

Jane M. Brokel, MSN, RN, is Executive Director of Care Management Institute for North Iowa Health Network, and a doctoral student at the University of Iowa.

Brenda K. Cobb, PhD, RN, is Assistant Professor at the School of Nursing, University of Alabama, Birmingham (formerly with the Center for Research on Chronic Illness, School of Nursing, University of North Carolina at Chapel Hill).

Sandra G. Funk, PhD, is Professor and Associate Director of the Center for Research on Chronic Illness, School of Nursing, University of North Carolina at Chapel Hill.

Sylvia Getman, MBA, is Marketing Specialist for North Iowa Mercy Health Center and Network.

Linda Goodwin, PhD, RN, is Nursing Informatics Scientist at the School of Nursing, Duke University.

Doreen J. Gudlin, MS, RN, is with the Department of Nursing, Mayo Medical Center.

Marcelline R. Harris, PhD, RN, is NLM Informatics Post-Doctoral Fellow, University of Minnesota.

Hal Hawkos, MBA, is Vice President of Information Systems for North Iowa Mercy Health Center and Network.

Carol L. Ireson, PhD, RN, is with the Center for Health Administration and Research, University of Kentucky.

Sally Kellum, MSN, RN-C, CCRN, is Clinical Coordinator for Hospital Informatics, Department of Veterans Affairs Medical Center, Durham, North Carolina.

Christine M. Kowalski, MS, RN, is Director of Clinical Information Management, Elder Health, Inc., Baltimore, Maryland.

Margaret Ross Kraft, MS, RN, is Chief, Spinal Cord Injury/Rehabilitation, Nursing Department of Veterans Affairs, The Edward Hines, Jr., Hospital, Hines, Illinois.

Barbara J. Lang, MSN, RN, is Project Manager, Information Resource Management Field Office, Department of Veterans Affairs, Hines, Illinois.

Eve L. Layman, MSN, RN, is Communication Resources Specialist, Center for Research on Chronic Illness, School of Nursing, University of North Carolina at Chapel Hill.

Russell C. McGuire, MS, RN, is Director of Clinical Services, Division of Home Services, Appalachian Regional Healthcare, Hazard, Kentucky.

Bobbie Owens-Vance (deceased), PhD, RN, was Chief of Nursing Services, Department of Veterans Affairs Medical Center, Atlanta, Georgia.

Cindy A. Scherb, MS, RN, is a doctoral student at the University of Iowa.

Larry P. Schumacher, MSN, RN, CNAA, is Chief Operating Officer and Senior Vice President of Clinical Integration for North Iowa Mercy Health Center and Network, and a doctoral student at the University of Iowa.

Tamara Schwichtenberg, RN, MS, is Clinical Information Specialist, North Iowa Mercy Health Center and Network.

Teresa Shellenbarger, DNSc, RN, CS, is Associate Professor of Nursing, Indiana University of Pennsylvania.

Mary Tatum, MSN, RN-C, is Nursing Informatics Coordinator, Department of Veterans Affairs Medical Center, Durham, North Carolina.

Jane A. Timm, MS, RN, is with the Department of Nursing, Mayo Medical Center.

Barbara Turner, PhD, RN, FAAN, is Associate Dean for Research, School of Nursing, Duke University.

Cathie L. Velotta, MSN, RN, is in Nursing Informatics, Department of Nursing, University of Kentucky Hospital.

Judith J. Warren, PhD, RN, FAAN, is a Clinical Nurse Researcher, University Hospital, and an Associate Professor, College of Nursing, University of Nebraska Medical Center, Omaha.

Jack Yensen, PhD, RN, is Webmaster, Virtual Nursing College and Faculty, Langara College, Vancouver, Canada.

Nashat Zuraikat, PhD, RN, is Professor of Nursing, Indiana University of Pennsylvania.

Printed in the United States
By Bookmasters